Praise for Payal Gidwani Tiwari

'Experience Payal's yoga techniques and you will thank me always.'

Malaika Arora Khan

'I feel like Payal has been not just a teacher, but someone who has been part of a journey with me. She is the instrument of change that helped me discover a more holistic approach to life. She is a very good trainer and has helped me do my best every single day.'

Rani Mukerji

'Payal is a wonderfully positive person who makes the experience of yoga and exercise so delightful. It was enlightenment to find a teacher like her.'

Jacqueline Fernandez

'Payal—whatever I say about her will never be enough! Her smile and absolutely loving nature got to me instantly. When I did my first yoga class with her and saw her in a yogic posture, I just knew I had found my yoga tutor for life. Her dedication to my body, her perseverance, loyalty, and commitment have helped me challenge my genes and transform my body to what it is today—from not being able to do five Suryanamaskars to doing 108 in the first five months is what Payal took me to. She has such a natural flair for yoga that even when she makes me do the toughest asana it becomes so easy! Her calming nature and the understanding she has shown towards my body is something I can never forget. Thank you Payal, thank you for yelling at me in every class but always with your loving smile. To me yoga is not a part of my life; it is my way of living and always will be!'

Kareena Kapoor

'I had been searching for a teacher who taught in a holistic manner and when I met Payal, I knew I had found my teacher. I love each and every session I take and feel brand new and charged when I practice yoga with her.'

Tamannaah Bhatia

'To be an excellent instructor you must be able to inspire and motivate your client. You must know how to push them and encourage them to willingly cross their limits of endurance. Payal does all this and more. I find her classes to be very challenging and look forward to them.'

Saif Ali Khan

'Payal's yoga is the best thing to have happened to me. It's been some time since I have been practicing this form of yoga and it has done wonders to my lifestyle and me. The entire process of learning yoga from Payal and her husband Manish has been very rewarding for me. Her form of yoga neither strains nor exhausts your body and mind. Apart from being physically fit and agile, my mind is completely at peace. I have been so satisfied that I have even introduced my children to yoga.'

Sridevi Kapoor

'I love working with Payal. She is a person who pushes you for sure but in a nice way, and to work out and sustain your workouts you need a gentle push. Her exercises make me feel great and more energetic as it is a beautiful blend of spiritualism and exercise.'

Priya Dutt

'I love working out with Payal because each workout seems absolutely different. I'm never completely tired after Payal's workout instead I'm completely charged for a brand new day. She is fun, encouraging and pushes you to *your* limits, not *hers*, and that is I think the deciding factor between a good yoga teacher and an excellent one. As for me, I'm always game to go back for more.'

Maria Goretti

'Payal introduced me to the world of yoga and thereby made a huge difference to my level of fi tness. She is very knowledgeable and sincere at the same time. On my first day, I found the postures very tough. However, thanks to her enthusiasm, I began enjoying the pain and the struggle that comes with being a beginner. Today I can't think of leaving and the credit for it goes to Payal.'

Tusshar Kapoor

'Payal has been super. Yoga and Payal have changed my life!'

Amrita Arora Ladak

'Payal is a dedicated and a reliable professional who is not only very passionate about what she does but also delivers results.'

Tulip Joshi

'Payal's Suryanamaskars are like magic. When I'm out of the country and have no time to train, I do 50 Suryanamaskars in the morning. It takes me just 20 minutes and I am able to maintain the bikini body through the holiday. It also helps to digest food faster and keeps my body free of toxins. Thank you Payal for showing me how to come back guilt free from my holidays!'

Zoa Morani

'If you are looking for overall well-being this book is for you. Yoga with Payal will do wonders for you physically and mentally.'

Shaheen Abbas

Body GODDESS

Also by the same author

From XL to XS

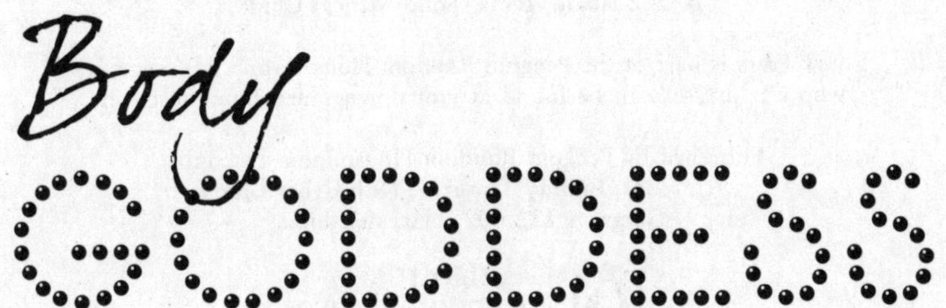

PAYAL GIDWANI TIWARI

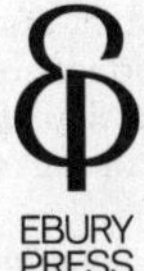

An imprint of Penguin Random House

EBURY PRESS

USA | Canada | UK | Ireland | Australia
New Zealand | India | South Africa | China

Ebury Press is part of the Penguin Random House group of companies whose addresses can be found at global.penguinrandomhouse.com

Published by Penguin Random House India Pvt. Ltd
7th Floor, Infinity Tower C, DLF Cyber City,
Gurgaon 122 002, Haryana, India

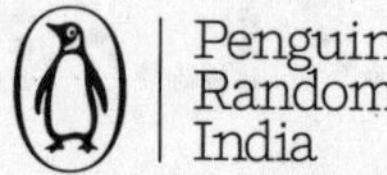

First published by Random House India 2015

10 9 8 7 6 5 4 3

The views and opinions expressed in this book are the author's own and the facts are as reported by her which have been verified to the extent possible, and the publishers are not in any way liable for the same.

ISBN 9788184000733

Typeset in Requiem Text by Manipal Digital Systems, Manipal
Printed at Replika Press Pvt. Ltd, India

www.penguin.co.in

To my husband Manish Tiwari and
son Sayaan Tiwari

Disclaimer: All the yoga exercises given in the book should be practiced under the guidance of an experienced teacher.

CONTENTS

FOREWORD

I love yoga. I do it to keep my mind calm and my body healthy. To feel good and stay happy. Since centuries, yoga is known as a good therapy for the mind, body, and soul. I feel there is nothing better than yoga to cope with today's demanding lifestyle. Not only do you feel positive when you do it, you also tend to think positive and glow from within.

I have been doing yoga since the past twelve years and I have become addicted to it. If I don't do it for even a day I feel I am missing something. It has become an inseparable part of my life. Yoga has also made me more energetic. I feel happy and healthy, and my body has become more flexible. I feel it is very important to be dedicated and do yoga regularly if you want to make the most of it. You have to be disciplined and take out the time. Whatever my schedule may be, I am willing to miss anything to take out time for yoga. You want to know why? Well, this is what keeps me going.

To be able to get the maximum benefits of yoga, you need a good teacher who can guide you in this extraordinary journey. I feel I am lucky to have a good teacher in Manish who has guided me properly, and Payal who motivates me constantly. In *Body Goddess: The Complete Guide on Yoga for Women*, Payal shares these extraordinary gems that can transform your lives too.

Thank you Payal and Manish for changing my life through yoga.

Keep up the good work.

Sridevi Kapoor
June 2015, Mumbai

INTRODUCTION

The journey continues

I have been doing yoga for more than a decade now and it is a way of life for me. Yoga as we know is an ancient form of meditation; an awareness practice that synchronizes the body, mind and breath. The word yoga is derived from the Sanskrit word 'yuj', which means 'to unify' or 'to yoke'. The practice has numerous physical and psychological benefits including improved strength, muscle tone, flexibility and joint mobility; better sleep, enhanced feelings of wellbeing, and relief from stress, anxiety and depression. Weight loss is the by-product of practicing yoga. The unique quality of yoga is that it works on the mind as well as the body and helps you stay focused on your goals. I learnt yoga from the most accomplished teachers, started Cosmic Fusion, my yoga studio where I continue to teach my students, and wrote *From XL to XS*, my debut book which was a smashing success thanks to my readers. In between I had a baby, gained weight, lost weight, and continue to practice yoga not only to keep my body slim but also to stay healthy and active.

Why does yoga hold an important place in my life? Well, to start with, it has been a life changing experience for me. It has helped me connect with my inner self that is so important in today's life. My tryst with yoga has continued over the years and with each passing year I feel the bond getting stronger. Moreover, I met my husband Manish, also a yoga teacher, during a yoga class and that was the icing on the cake. It has been an amazing journey and you all have been an important part of it. I am thankful to all my readers who read my book and to those who found the time to write to me sharing their stories, problems and seeking advice. In *Body Goddess,* I have talked about and shared solutions to issues faced by my students, readers as well my own personal struggles.

Fat or Fit

I often wonder and wish we all looked like Heidi Klum or Naomi Campbell but we Indians have a distinctive body structure unique to us. We have our own distinctive bone structure, shapes and sizes and, we should all be proud of it. We are gifted with a range of complexions, skin tones, hair types as well as body structures with apple, pear, hour glass, wine glass being the most common ones. In my first book *From XL to XS*, I had discussed these at length and what we can do to maintain the ideal body weight with different body shapes. Believe me, it really helps if you are aware of your weak spots and areas where you are prone to put on weight. Knowing that I am apple shaped, I keep a watch on my stomach where I have a tendency to put on weight very quickly.

The other day I went to buy my monthly grocery from the nearby supermarket in Bombay. There were rows and rows of colourful, attractive packets of biscuits, namkeens, snacks, noodles, chocolates and treats. My four-year-old son was wide eyed, excited and jumping about in excitement. If a child can get tempted so, what about us? The truth is, in today's world we are spoilt for choice. There are dozens of varieties and brands of everything, and believe me they all look fetching at first glance. To resist and keep away from packaged products which have preservatives among other things is getting increasingly difficult. How many times have you said, 'I'll just have one'? But does it ever stop at one? The answer is most likely no. I am reminded of the story of my friend Tara Kulkarni.

When we were growing up, Tara was clearly one of the fittest amongst us. She was a swimmer, model and in her twenties led a very active social life. She got married at the age of twenty nine and had a baby at thirty two. At thirty five when I bumped into her I could not recognize Tara. I was shocked. She seemed a faint shadow of the person I knew. We got talking and she told me how she had gotten really busy with her job and the baby, and had no time to swim or manage her lifestyle. She had stopped exercising and was eating whatever came her way, mostly ready to eat things. She was more than twenty kilos overweight and looked burnt out. When I was standing in the queue to pay my bill I could see many more Taras in front of me.

Yes, we are getting fatter. Much more than before. Simply looking around is enough for us to realize this. Our mums and grandmums were fit and had lesser health conditions even with no workouts and dietitians. They led an active life, ate home-cooked and fresh foods and led a routine life. This is not the life we lead. It is very easy for us to forget our roots and the basics of nutrition when we are wide-eyed and always tempted to try out the new flavours launched in the junk food segment, the healthy 'diet' foods that the packaging almost shouts out at us and the increasing stress on eating out while avoiding home-cooked food due to various reasons. To top all this, most of us have busy professional lives which often include late or erratic work hours and a lot of travelling. Being a homemaker is no mean feat either. It is equally tough to be a good housewife, managing the needs of everybody in the family. All this has resulted in an imbalance in our bodies resulting in weight issues coupled with health issues like diabetes, thyroid, heart ailments, PCOS and so on. There is no escape from these unless we understand our bodies and learn to balance our lifestyle with exercise and dietary changes. No wonder there has been a rapid increase in the number of obese people in the country, and shockingly in all age groups even children, teenagers and people in their twenties. In fact, according to a recent study conducted by doctors from India's National Diabetes, Obesity and Cholesterol Foundation, this is more prevalent in the affluent living in the metros of India.

Growing health issues

How often do you go to a doctor in a year? From common colds, viral infections to other regular health issues? This is even more common for children and I remember how I used to hate going to the clinics and hospitals while growing up. Now even busy globetrotters, housewives, working professionals face the same issues. Every summer and rainy season we hear of a fresh onslaught of dengue, malaria, typhoid, jaundice, conjunctivitis and so on. The list is endless. Besides these seasonal diseases, women are increasingly getting affected by thyroid, diabetes, PCOS, arthritis, back aches, PMS, infertility and premature ageing among other things. Why do you think this is happening?

I have been working with women of all age groups and I have been noticing how the number of incidences of diseases which were not so common few years ago have been steadily going up. One of the most common reasons that experts point out is the lack of immunity coupled with bad lifestyle habits especially lack of exercise and unbalanced diet. Who wants to stay in bed and miss all the fun? Life is precious and like they say the time gone past never returns. We all want to enjoy life, be happy and feel good from within. In *Body Goddess*, I want to talk about how you can stay healthy and look good, and how yoga can help you achieve that.

I have often heard women even in their twenties or younger grumbling about how they do not have the energy and feel tired all the time. Seema Verma, a sixteen-year-old college student, always complained about feeling low and avoided going out with her friends. She felt left out and unhappy about not being able to do things a regular girl of her age did. She was slim, looked healthy, even fit. When her parents took her for a thorough medical examination, she was diagnosed with juvenile diabetes. And this is not an isolated case. These instances are getting much more common as we deal with our modern lifestyle.

In the course of this book, I will show you how you can not only achieve a slim and fit body but also a healthy one. To enjoy life to the fullest, have the energy and stamina to do multiple things, you don't only need a slim body. What you really need is a healthy body that makes you look good at the same time. So here's what I recommend as a step by step approach to a lifetime of health and fitness:

- Know your body shape
  Find out what body shape you are and learn to play to your strengths.
- Accept that you are different
  Stop comparing yourself with others as this will get you nowhere. With acceptance comes confidence and grace.
- Work on your weak spots
  Just as it is important to know your strengths, it is equally important to know what you need to work on. Once you know if it is your stomach or your thighs, you can plan your workout accordingly.
- Never ignore a health condition that you might have
  Indian women have a tendency to ignore their health issues until it becomes unbearable. Listen to your body and take medical advice early on to get back on track sooner.
- Aim for holistic remedies
  Health is a combination of a lot of things and exercise is only a part of it. Meditation, diet, sleep are also key for your health and that is why I always recommend a holistic solution for lasting good health.
- Exercise regularly and balance your diet accordingly.
- Disciple and routine is the key to staying fit and slim and it rings true for exercise and diet as well.

In Part Two of the book I will show you how we can go about this and lead a healthy, happy, and beautiful life.

Why this second book?

I wrote *From XL to XS* to share what I had learnt from my teachers and what I had imbibed while teaching my students. Most importantly, I wanted to break the myths surrounding yoga that it is boring, a static form of exercise, only for older people, does not help lose weight, difficult to do, and so on. I felt I should clear the air and share my experiences. I'm delighted I have been able to achieve some of what I set out to do with *From XL to XS*.

I have been flooded with queries and feedback after *From XL to XS* was published.

Sharon Randhawa wrote to me from the UK about her struggles with losing the nagging last few kilos; Dinana Vineet Sharma from Kolkata wrote to me saying she gifted the book to all her friends; Sayyeda Sumaira Savaiz from Lahore, Pakistan wanted to start doing yoga after coming across *From XL to XS;* Alisha Ramdaw from South Africa was interested in how to get a toned as well as a slim body through yoga.

So why this second book? While the focus of *From XL to XS* was weight loss, *Body Goddess* stresses on the overall health and well-being for a woman. To be honest, it was born out of my interactions with my readers and the questions I have been receiving. Women facing various health issues would write to me about possible solutions and if there were any yoga exercises they could do. In this book I have delved deeper into the basics of yoga that make it such a holistic and useful practice. I talk about Chakras, Kriyas, Pranayam, Asanas, as well as Suryanamaskar. In the different chapters of the book, I talk about the various health issues that women face at different stages of their lives. Yoga as we know is a vast treasure trove of knowledge with solutions for health conditions ranging from PCOD, thyroid, diabetes, menopause and so on. I have included workouts and exercises for all these as well as one basic workout for weight loss. I hope you enjoy reading the book as much as I did putting it together.

I have always believed that what makes you look good is not only a slim body but a fit and healthy one. I want you to love and own your body, listen to it, understand it, and follow what suits your lifestyle. There is no substitute for the inner glow that comes only from wholesome well-being, and that is what I hope you will achieve after reading and practising what has been laid out in the book. The unmistakable glow of a Body Goddess.

PART ONE

CHAKRAS: THE WHEELS OF LIFE ENERGY

Does the word 'chakra' sound familiar to you? You must have heard it on TV shows or read about it in newspapers and magazines. In this chapter I want to talk about some fundamentals of yoga which will help us understand our bodies better. Chakra is one of them.

How are chakras relevant to yoga? Chakras are energy centres in our body which are awakened and channelized when we do yoga. The better we understand and utilize the energy that is stored up within our body, the better the results of yoga workouts will be. Before we go into Part Two of the book and discuss workout regimes, I feel it is important to learn the basics.

We all know how the ancient Indian healing systems have made a comeback not only in India but across the world. There is a stress on going back to our roots and rediscovering our past. Whether it is Ayurveda or healing medicinal oil massages in spas, we all have taken to it like fish to water. There is an ever increasing stress on words like natural, organic, and green. Every active, outgoing, contemporary woman wants to try it and feel the difference.

You know how home and work pressure, nine-to-five jobs, strained relationships, family problems, health issues, and stressful lives have become the norm for most of us. In this fast-paced mobile world of social networking, Twitter, Facebook, and virtual identities, don't you at times feel the need to slow down a little and think about yourself at times? This is the reason why your need to understand what chakras are and how they have an impact in our lives.

Now, you might say, I have a vague idea but don't exactly know what it is. Don't worry; I'll explain it to you. First of all let me tell you that understanding chakras isn't rocket science. It is neither a magic spell that you can't learn nor a puzzle that you can't solve. Chakras are simply seven spinning wheels or energy centres, positioned between the top of your head and the end of your spine (see picture below). Its healing involves channelizing the body's forces of energy. It is believed that all sorts of weaknesses—physical as well as emotional can be cured by the energy field within and around our body. Unlike most modern-day therapies, the focus of this system is to principally revive and rejuvenate your life, inside out. The approach is more holistic and long-term.

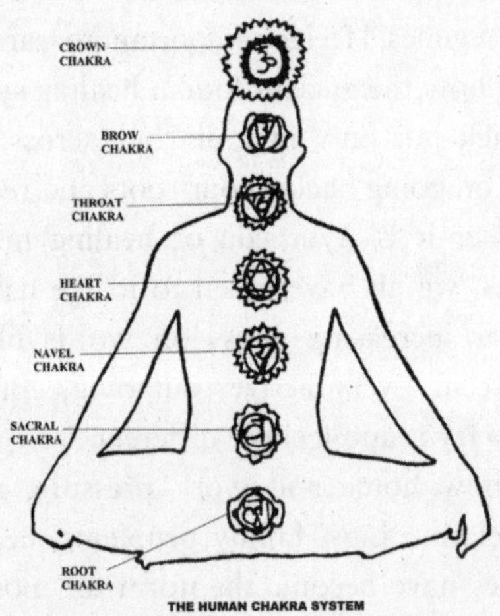

THE HUMAN CHAKRA SYSTEM

UNDERSTANDING CHAKRAS

Shimla, Mussoorie, Darjeeling, Ooty, and Mahabaleshwar—you must have been to at least one of these places on your honeymoon or summer holidays. Right? What is the first thing that comes to your mind when you think about these destinations? I am sure you remember the lush green surroundings and the serene beauty. Now picture this—you are on a vacation and staying in a multi-storied hotel in the vicinity of scenic mountains. Sounds romantic, doesn't it?

It is obvious that before choosing a room, you'd like to take a look at the view from different floors. You climb the stairs and reach the room on the first floor. When you open the windows you realize that you can see the mountains, but the noisy market below disturbs your peace of mind. You then decide to take the elevator and take a look at the other rooms. With every floor you realize that the sight becomes clearer and the din from the market settles down. The seventh floor offers you the best vantage point. You not only get a majestic view of the mountains, but it is also be the quietest. If there's no fog clouding the windows, you'll be able to see a panoramic view of the hill station from this floor.

For a minute, take a deep breath and just think about your own body—you'll realize that it's exactly like the hotel. You'd ask me, so what's the connection between my body, chakras, and a hotel? Interestingly, the seven windows on each floor are like the seven chakras of your body. Our complex lifestyles often cause a distorted and unclear perspective of our lives. Like the fog on the windows, these complexities blur our vision. The higher we go and get to know the various chakras, our understanding becomes clearer and better—peaceful surroundings and an all-encompassing viewpoint helps us in knowing the outer as well as the inner self.

THE HUMAN CHAKRA SYSTEM

Now that your basic concept is clear, let's discuss the human chakra system in detail. There is more to your body than just the material self. Two aspects govern it—the visible and the invisible. The visible part is what you can see and notice while the invisible part remains hidden from your physical senses. The chakras are such unseen whirlpools of energy within our bodies that need to be awakened. Now you'll say—if something cannot be seen, why trouble myself with it? How can some invisible force affect my life?

I know a lot of questions are popping up in your mind. Well yes, mind—can you see it? Emotions, faith, joy, pain, love—you cannot see any of these either, but you do believe in their existence, don't you? Even if you can't touch or see them you can definitely feel them. Similarly, chakras are invisible but once awakened you can feel the change they can bring in your life.

Chakra in Sanskrit stands for the 'wheel'—literally meaning the sphere of a man's energy. Out of the innumerable chakras only seven are vital. These are like different coloured flowers with varying number of petals or nadis. The petals can be of any number from four to thousand. Constantly rotating, they act as power magnets. As we move from the lower level of the body to the crown of our heads, the number of petals increases. The midpoint of each flower-like chakra possesses an important energy channel, sushumma, which connects all the chakras to each other. You can picture a string of seven pearls connected by a nylon thread to understand it. The thread is the sushumma and the pearls are the chakras.

IMPORTANCE OF CHAKRAS

I am sure by now you have a fair idea about chakras. But just grasping the theoretical aspect isn't enough. Since your busy, hectic life often leaves you fatigued, you need to know the importance of chakras to recharge your energies and channelize your true potential. To start with I feel you need to know what is best for you in order to achieve it. Imagine a red apple—it might appear fresh and ripe from the outside, but its inner core is rotten. Would you be able to eat it? Your body is important but your inner self, both mental and spiritual, too needs to be cleansed of impurities. Only then will you be able to enjoy true health. To properly deal with your problems, you need to have a fair idea about how to activate and purify chakras. In the next section, I'll discuss in detail the seven primary chakras and ways to energize them.

THE 7 PRINCIPAL CHAKRAS

Do you know how many chakras are mentioned in traditional writings? Make a guess? 88,000! Surprising, isn't it? Fortunately, you don't need to bother yourself with all that information. Out of this huge number, only 40 secondary ones are considered important. But, for the proper working of your body, mind, and soul, you need to know only seven:

1. Root or Muladhara Chakra
2. Sacral or Svadhistana Chakra
3. Navel or Manipura Chakra
4. Heart or Anahata Chakra
5. Throat or Visuddha Chakra
6. Brow or Ajna Chakra
7. Crown or Sahasrara Chakra

Based on their position in our bodies, the seven chakras can be classified into three sub-groups:

a. Lower—Root and Sacral Chakras
b. Middle—Navel, Heart, and Throat Chakras
c. Higher—Brow and Crown Chakras

Now that you know the names of the seven chakras, let me explain each one to you in detail.

1. ROOT or MULADHARA CHAKRA

This is the first energy centre located at the end of your spine, near the tailbone. It holds the entire system strong and steady as a foundation pillar and is therefore placed at the lowest level. You can think of it as the roots of a tree. If the roots are not nourished or watered properly would the tree grow? If it is cut, the tree would soon become lifeless and eventually die. Like a tree needs its roots for survival, you need Muladhara Chakra for the proper functioning of your body. In order to maintain balance in your life, you need to work on this base chakra.

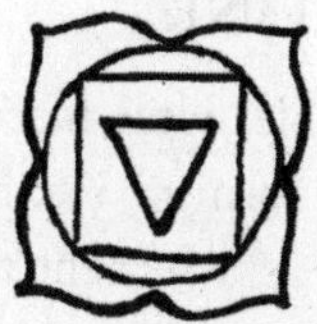

Figure 1: Root Chakra

Due to its close contact with Mother Earth, it is associated with the colour red. It gives an earthly firmness and a solid ground on which you can build your life. Its symbol is a four-petal lotus flower, which represents the four directions of earth–north, east, west, and south. For a better understanding, think of it as the four tyres of a car. If one wheel is missing, the car would not move. As you can see in the figure, there is a downward pointing triangle in its centre. This triangle symbolizes the downward force which connects it with the earth.

If your root chakra is balanced, you'll feel satisfied and experience stability and inner strength in your life. It is associated with the adrenal gland and its energy affects your DNA, feet, legs, hips, ovaries, spine, and vagina. On the other hand, if your chakra is jammed, you'll lack emotional and physical firmness. You'll be easily irritated, infuriated and feel anxiety and insecurity. Rage, violence, and sadness are indications of the absence of self-trust.

Interestingly, this Root Chakra is also the home of Kundalini. Now you'd ask, what's that? Sure, I'm coming to that.

WHAT IS KUNDALINI?

Kundalini is the invisible, vital force lying dormant within the root chakra in the form of inexhaustible, coiled energy. It is usually visualized as a serpent twisted into three and a half coils, spiraling near the tailbone. The awakening of this serpent and manifestation of its powers is the primary aim of Kundalini Yoga.

The purpose is to awaken and then arouse the serpent, in the form of dynamic Shakti, the Mother Goddess. When she's ready to unfold, it is believed she ascends through the other chakras, to unite the crown of our head with Shiva, the Universal Father encircling the cosmos.

Among the innumerable energies surrounding our body, Kundalini is the most subtle, having the highest spiritual dimension. Once awakened, it spontaneously starts balancing all the other energies and stabilizes all the aspects of our life and growth. Self-awareness has always been the improbable goal of all cultures and civilizations of the world. Kundalini Yoga is a way to attain it. If you want to try it, make sure you do it only under the guidance of an experienced teacher or an expert.

ACTIVATING AND ENERGIZING THE ROOT CHAKRA

Do you often experience any of the following?

- Anger
- Backache
- Fatigue
- Fear

- o Self-consciousness
- o Stomach disorders
- o Tension

If the answer is yes, your root chakra is congested and needs to be opened up. There are various therapies that can help to activate and purify it.

- Aroma therapy

Who doesn't like nice fragrances? Perfume your life with any of these aroma oils—black pepper, cedar, clove, ginger, rosemary, or wood. You can also buy aroma candles available freely now or put a few drops of your preferred oil into an aroma lamp and light it in your bedroom or living room. The aromas help to stimulate the chakra and bring the balance back.

- Colour therapy

The root chakra can be stimulated by a pure, bright shade of red. You can wear a sexy red dress, or have foods rich in iron and potassium. Consuming fruits like cherry, plum, and water melon can prove beneficial. You can also have a glass of apple juice mixed with beetroot, tomatoes or strawberries to feel the difference.

- Gemstone therapy

Gemstones are in vogue nowadays. A lot more people want to try it out. Agate, blood jasper, garnet, hematite, red coral, or ruby can be used to stimulate your chakra, and also add oomph to your style statement.

• Nature therapy

Spending time in nature's lap is in itself a beautiful experience. Watching the rosy sunrise or sunset can be truly heart-warming. To activate the root chakra—sit on the ground and breathe in the fragrance of mother earth. Gardening and pottery can also be developed as a hobby.

• Sound therapy

Nature is an abundant source of musical rhythms. Being close to the environment can be beneficial as its various sounds can inspire healing. Soothing music, mantras and chants can be used to heal your chakra.

• Yoga therapy

Hatha Yoga, an ancient form of yoga, and Kundalini Yoga are primarily used to energize the root chakra. You can try Tadasana—tree pose, Paschimottanasana—seated forward bend, Setubandhasana—bridge pose, and Uttanasana—standing forward bend. (For details refer to the chapter on Exercises.)

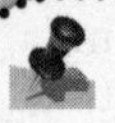

ROOT or MULADHARA CHAKRA

Colour	Fiery red
Element	Earth
Sense	Smell
Associated Gland	Adrenal
Principle	Survival, security, and stability
Location	Base of spine, tailbone
Symbol	A four-petal lotus

(*Cont.*)

Bodily Association	DNA, anus, blood, bones, feet, legs, hips, ovaries, penis, rectum, spine, teeth, and vagina
Imbalances	Anxiety, shyness, insecurity, cowardice, anemia, fatigue, lower back pain, nerve pain, depression, too much self-consciousness
Stimulants	Meditation, foot massage, gardening, and pottery. Red coloured foods and drinks. Red gemstones, red clothing, and red oils

2. SACRAL or SVADHISTANA CHAKRA

The second energy centre is the most feminine of all, located just below your navel, near the lower abdomen. It is the centre of your creativity, desires, emotions, grace, pleasure, and sexual vitality. As we climb the ladder of Chakras, the second one transforms into a liquid form in contrast to the first solid, earthy chakra. Like roots need water for survival, this nourishing chakra provides the root chakra with vitality. It is in a constant state of producing new life.

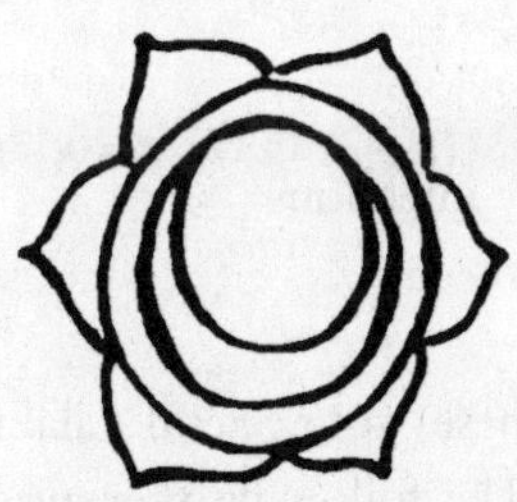

Figure 2: Spleen Chakra

Since its element is water, it represents change, movement, and mobility in your life. It also has purifying properties. Sacral Chakra is associated with orange colour and is thought to be the actual seat of Shakti—in the form of creative energy. Its symbol is a six-petal lotus flower, which is related to the moon. Like the moon affects tides and ebbs on earth, this energy centre affects your ever-changing, fluid life energy.

If your Sacral Chakra is functioning properly, you'll feel self-confident and experience emotional balance and stability. It is associated with the ovaries as well as the gonads. Its energy affects your bladder, blood, kidneys, lymph, reproductive organs, and spleen. If you successfully eliminate addiction, fear, and anxiety, you'll be able to purify this chakra and block feelings like lack of self-esteem, emotional paralysis, and sexual issues.

ACTIVATING AND ENERGIZING THE SACRAL CHAKRA

Do you often experience any of the following?

- Unhappiness
- Frustration
- Lack of sexual desire
- Jealousy
- Menstrual pain
- Bladder and Kidney infections
- Suppressed emotions

If you face any of these, your Sacral Chakra is blocked and needs to be cured. The following therapies can help you in activating and energizing it.

• Aroma therapy

You can mix a few drops of bitter orange with jojoba oil and massage the area just below your navel. You can also take a warm bath with a few drops of vanilla or sandalwood oil to activate this chakra.

• Colour therapy

A clear shade of vibrant orange energizes the second chakra. Wearing orange clothes, or eating carrots, oranges, pumpkin, apricots, and crab can prove beneficial. You can also place orange flowers in your living room.

• Gemstone therapy

Carnelian, Moonstone, and Sunstone can be used for meditation. You can also add a dash of colour to your trinkets by wearing any of these gemstones as earrings or necklaces.

• Nature therapy

Take a walk by the ocean on a moonlit night. It will not only be refreshing but also very soothing. On a full moon night, you can spend time contemplating while looking outside the window. Sounds romantic, doesn't it? Well it heals your Sacral chakra as well.

• Sound therapy

Any type of soothing and melodious music can energize this chakra. You can also listen to the sound of chirping birds or rhythmic waves of the sea.

• Yoga therapy

Tantra Yoga is chiefly used to invigorate the Sacral Chakra. You can try Ardha Matsyendrasana—twisted pose, Bhujangasana—cobra posture, and Trikonasana—triangle pose. (See the chapter on Exercises.)

SACRAL or SVADHISTANA CHAKRA

Colour	Orange
Element	Water
Sense	Taste
Associated Gland	Gonads and Ovaries
Principle	The right to feel. Creative reproduction of being
Location	Lower abdomen, below the navel
Symbol	A six-petal lotus
Bodily Association	Kidneys, bladder, pelvic girdle, reproductive organs, blood, lymph, sperm, and spleen
Imbalances	Anger, depression, frustration, jealousy, painful menstruation, emotional suppression, eating disorders, alcohol and drug abuse, allergies, lack of sexual desire, and impotence
Spleen Stimulants	Walking by the sea on a moonlit night, hot aromatic bath, water sports, massage, orange coloured food and drinks, orange gemstones, and oils

3. NAVEL or MANIPURA CHAKRA

The third chakra is located below the breastbone and behind the stomach. While the second chakra represents change and movement, this energy centre is dense and depicts stability.

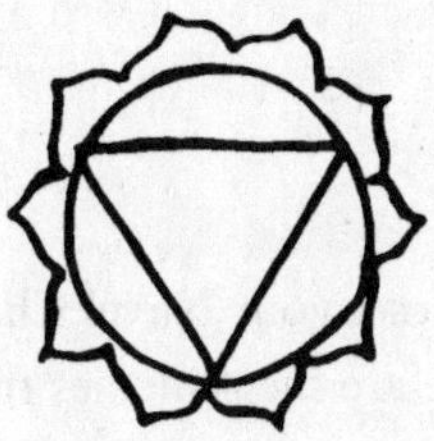

Figure 3: Navel Chakra

As this chakra represents the sun, it is associated with the element of fire. It represents clarity of thought, ego, self-esteem, power, light, warmth as well as purification. It is associated with yellow colour and purifies the desires of the lower chakras. Its symbol is a ten-petal lotus flower, with a downward pointing triangle which signifies fire.

When your Navel Chakra is functioning properly, you'll feel inner harmony, peace, and wisdom. It would be easy for you to accept yourself, as you are. It is associated with the pancreas and its energy affects your digestive system, abdomen, stomach, liver, gallbladder, nervous system, and spleen. To be able to energize this chakra you need to eliminate lack of motivation, feeling of powerlessness, and low self-esteem.

ACTIVATING AND ENERGIZING THE NAVEL CHAKRA

Do you often experience any of the following:

- Aggression
- Lack of will power

- Lack of self-esteem
- Negativity
- Constipation
- Diabetes
- Vulnerability

If you face any of these, your Navel Chakra needs treatment as it is blocked. Here are the remedies that I recommend:

- Aroma therapy

You can use any of these oils for emotional balance and to take care of your digestive system—rose, sandalwood, lemon, peppermint, lavender, ginger, chamomile, or frankincense. You can put a few drops in water, before taking a bath.

- Colour therapy

You can wear yellow clothes or use yellow bed covers, cushions and curtains to brighten up your room. A bouquet of yellow sunflowers, candle-lit dinner, and sitting by the fireside can also help.

- Gemstone therapy

Amber, Citrine, Topaz, and Yellow Jasper are some beautiful gemstones that you can use in the form of bracelets. It is important that the stone is in touch with your skin.

- Nature therapy

Open your curtains and welcome the sunshine into your bedroom. You can also enjoy walking or lying down on a beach on a sunny day.

• Sound therapy

Harmonious and fiery orchestral music can enhance this energy centre. You can also practice chanting the mantra Ram to awaken this chakra.

• Yoga therapy

Karma Yoga is beneficial for this chakra. You can try Dhanurasana—bow posture, Bhujangasana—cobra pose, and Ardha Pada Hastasana—leg lifts. (See the chapter on Exercises for details.)

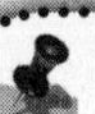

NAVEL or MANIPURA CHAKRA

Colour	Yellow-golden
Element	Fire
Sense	Sight
Associated Gland	Pancreas
Principle	Shaping of things—personal power
Location	About two finger-breadths above the navel
Symbol	A ten-petal lotus
Bodily Association	Abdomen, digestive system, liver, gallbladder, spleen, nervous system, and back
Imbalances	Inner restlessness, manipulation, struggle for survival, digestive problems, diabetes, constipation, nervousness, and poor memory
Root Stimulants	Mind puzzles, sunbath, detoxification diets, yellow food and drinks, clothing and gemstones. Also using yellow oils such as lemon or sandalwood

4. HEART or ANAHATA CHAKRA

The fourth chakra is associated with compassion and an all-encompassing love. It is located near the heart as you would have already guessed by now. Interestingly, it can work as a channel for divine love. Located centrally, it is the meeting point of lower and higher chakras. While the first three energy centres represent the self, the fourth chakra represents relationships.

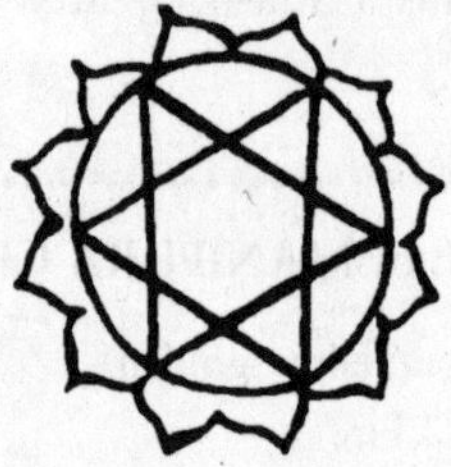

Figure 4: Heart Chakra

You need air to ignite fire; hence this chakra's associated element is air. Interestingly, air also signifies life-breath or prana, which is an important component of the Human Chakra System. It is usually represented by the colour green, but sometimes pink or golden may also be used. Its symbol is a twelve-petal lotus flower, within which lie two triangles– upward as well as downward facing, forming a fascinating star. The two triangles depict the union of the feminine and the masculine forces.

Our capability to empathize as well as sympathize depends on this chakra. If this energy centre is functioning properly, you'll yearn for deep intimate contact, and fear separation. You will also experience unconditional love, beauty, harmony, and forgiveness. It is associated with the thymus and its energy affects your heart, blood, circulatory system, skin, upper back, and lower area of lungs. If you can cast off depression, indifference, and the fear of rejection, you'll be able to successfully purify this chakra.

ACTIVATING AND ENERGIZING THE HEART CHAKRA

Do you often experience any of the following:

- Loneliness
- Problems with sustaining relationships
- Feeling unloved
- Heart issues
- Respiratory problems
- Allergies
- Inability to love others or yourself

If you face any of these, your heart chakra is dysfunctional. This can be treated via various methods.

- Aroma therapy

You can use oils like rose, ylang ylang, rosewood, jasmine, eucalyptus, and chamomile. You can put a few drops of any of these oils on a handkerchief and breathe into it whenever you feel like.

- Colour therapy

The colour of green bushes and forests can give you a soothing effect. You can revamp your home with green plants and décor. Wearing green clothes or having veggies can also enhance the effect of this chakra.

- Gemstone therapy

Emerald, Green Amber, Jade, Kunzite, Rose Quartz, and Tourmaline are the stones associated with healing properties. You can place any of these on the centre of your chest and meditate for a few minutes.

- Nature therapy

A walk through the countryside is an enriching experience. You can go to any park or garden for a morning or an evening walk. The pink-violet evening sky can also help you in energizing this chakra. Let go of the past and things that hurt you. Accept yourself and forgo negative feelings.

- Sound therapy

Classical or meditative music can prove helpful as well as chanting the mantra Yam to activate this chakra.

- Yoga therapy

You can try Bhakti Yoga. These asanas would definitely help—Ushtrasana, Matsyasana, and Gomukhasana. (See the chapter on Exercises for details.)

HEART or ANAHATA CHAKRA

Colour	Green, pink, or golden
Element	Air
Sense	Touch
Associated Gland	Thymus
Principle	Devotion, self-abandon, and an all-encompassing love
Location	Chest, near the heart
Symbol	A twelve-petal lotus
Bodily Association	Heart, upper back, lower lungs, blood, circulatory system, and skin
Imbalances	Breathing disorder, heart and breast cancer, high blood pressure, chest and muscular pain, and passivity
Root Stimulants	Nature walks, trekking, spending time with family and friends, wearing green clothes, eating leafy vegetables, using green oils, and gemstones

5. THROAT or VISUDDHA CHAKRA

The fifth energy centre is located at the base of your throat. It is the core of your creative expression and communication. As you move upwards towards the higher chakras, you'll realize that the self becomes more and more distant. Since we all are social animals, it is extremely important to communicate, be it verbally or non-verbally. Chakras operate by means of vibrations and interestingly, sound too is produced through vibrations.

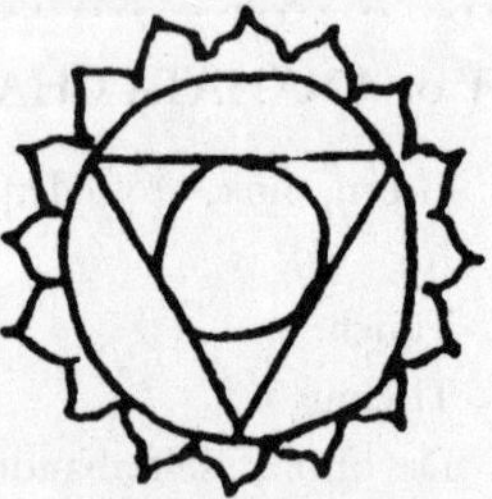

Figure 5: Throat Chakra

Its element ether or sound represents seen as well as unseen vibrations. Associated with pale blue, silver or greenish-blue colour, its symbol is a sixteen-petal lotus flower, with a circle in the centre representing a full moon. The sixteen petals contain all the 16 vowels of Sanskrit.

If this chakra is functioning properly, you'll feel active, wise, and independent. It is associated with thyroid and its energy affects your neck, throat, ears, voice, trachea, upper lungs, arms, and jaw. If you can let go of shyness and stiffness you can eliminate uncertainty, lack of confidence, and self-built walls.

ACTIVATING AND ENERGIZING THE THROAT CHAKRA

Do you often experience any of the following?

- Difficulty in communicating with others
- Shyness
- Lack of self-esteem
- Dental issues
- Thyroid problems
- Sore throat or tonsillitis
- Habit of telling lies

If you face any of these, your throat chakra is blocked and needs the following therapies.

- Aroma therapy

Oils which can heal this chakra are tea tree, peppermint, eucalyptus, rosewood, and lavender. You can have a sauna bath using lavender or tea tree oil

- Colour therapy

You can place blue vases and candle holders in your room. Blue towels, mattresses, blankets, upholstery and clothes can also be used to enhance your throat chakra.

- Gemstone therapy

Turquoise, Aquamarine, and Topaz are beautiful stones. You can carry it off in style by teaming it with your favourite top or kurti.

- Nature therapy

Lie down on the ground and gaze at the endless blue sky. Sit by a beautiful beach and enjoy the cool breeze while reading your favourite book.

- Sound therapy

Music rich in high tones and meditative rhythms can be harmonizing. You can also chant the mantra HAM for it.

- Yoga therapy

Mantra Yoga can be practised through asanas like Sarvangasana, Halasana, and Matsyasana. You can read about them in detail in the chapter on Asanas.

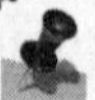

THROAT or VISUDDHA CHAKRA

Colour	Pale blue, silver, greenish blue
Element	Ether
Sense	Hearing
Associated Gland	Thyroid
Principle	Resonance of being—our ability to communicate
Location	Base of the throat
Symbol	A sixteen-petal lotus
Bodily Association	Neck, throat, ears, voice, trachea, upper lungs, oesophagus, arms, and jaw
Imbalances	Thyroid imbalance, infections, flu, fever; mouth, tongue, jaw infection, mood swings, hormonal imbalance, and menopause
Root Stimulants	Poetry and artistic hobbies, meaningful conversations, blue food and drinks. Blue gemstones, clothing, and oils

6. BROW or AJNA CHAKRA

The sixth chakra is located between the eyebrows, at the centre of the forehead. Also called the third eye, this energy centre depicts sight, creative visualization, sixth sense, intuition, perception, and psychic ability. The most fascinating aspect of this chakra is that it is not based on any particular element and affects all the senses—sensory as well as extrasensory.

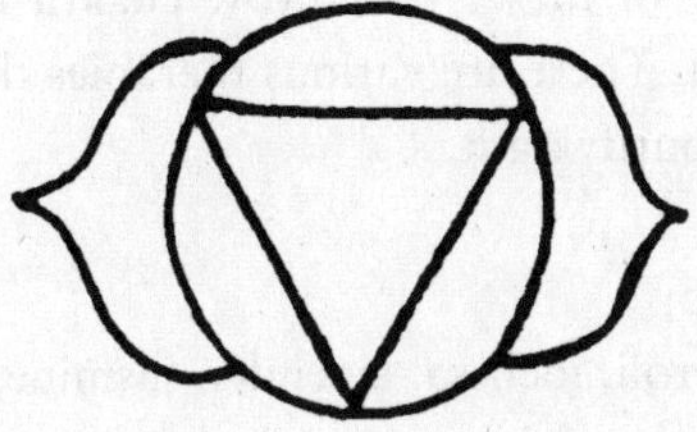

Figure 6: Brow Chakra

Its symbol is a ninety-six-petal lotus flower, divided into two main parts containing 48 petals each. If your brow chakra is dysfunctional, you'll experience blindness in seeing the truth and the inability to comprehend reality. It is associated with the pituitary glands and affects your face, eyes, ears, nose, sinuses, and central nervous system. Meditation, rational thought, intellectual cognition, and knowledge can help in attaining harmony and will also balance this chakra.

ACTIVATING AND ENERGIZING THE BROW CHAKRA

Do you often any of the following?

- Panic attacks
- Lack of concentration
- Lack of faith in yourself
- Headache or sinus
- Learning disability
- Eyesight or hearing problems
- Dizziness

If you face any of these, your brow chakra is clogged and needs treatment. There are various therapies that can help in activating and purifying it.

- Aroma therapy

Lemongrass, neroli, melissa, lavender, jasmine, frankincense, and elemi are some of the aroma oils that you can use. A great aromatherapy massage would be wonderful for your chakra healing.

- Colour therapy

Transparent indigo has a cleansing effect and provides clarity and calmness. Revamp your home with dark blue curtains and bed sheets. You can also wear dark blue T-shirts with a pair of slim-fit jeans.

- Gemstone therapy

Lapis Lazuli, Blue Sapphire, Sodalite, and Azurite are the best stones to stimulate this chakra. A sapphire pendant can really enhance your fashionable clothes.

- Nature therapy

Looking at the starry night sky can be an awesome experience to connect with your energy centre.

- Sound therapy

New Age music can soothe and relax your mind. You can also chant the mantra KSHAM for it.

• Yoga therapy

Jnana Yoga and Yantra Yoga are beneficial. You can try Sarvangasana and Matsyasana. For in-depth analysis refer to the chapter on Asanas.

BROW or AJNA CHAKRA

Colour	Indigo, yellow, yellow-green, violet
Sense	Sight, sound, smell, taste, touch, and extrasensory perception
Associated Gland	Pituitary
Principle	Knowledge of being—the third eye
Location	Centre of the forehead, between the eyebrows
Symbol	A ninety-six-petal lotus
Bodily Association	Face, eyes, ears, nose, sinuses, central nervous system, and cerebellum
Imbalances	Hyperactivity, PMS, hormonal imbalance, intellectual arrogance, materialistic desires, muddled thinking
Root Stimulants	Meditation, star-gazing. Indigo or blue coloured foods like some berries and drinks. Blue gemstones like Sapphire, clothes, and oils

7. CROWN or SAHASRARA CHAKRA

The seventh chakra, also called the seat of enlightenment, is located at the top of the head. It is the centre of your thoughts, knowledge, and wisdom. It unites in itself all the energies of the lower chakras. This energy centre has dual movements: downward—from top to bottom within the body and upwards moving from the head beyond the visible world.

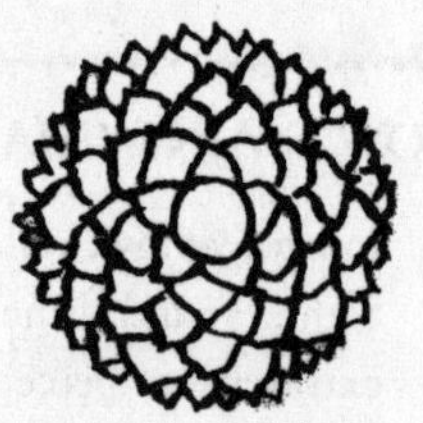

Figure 3: Crown Chakra

Having no physical boundary—that is the reverse of root chakra and represents concentration, devotion, and oneness with the Omnipresent Being. Associated with three colours–violet, white, and gold, its symbol is a thousand-petal lotus flower. Since 0 represents infinity, so do the 1000 petals. If this chakra is blocked, it may cause depression, confusion, alienation, boredom, and apathy. It is associated with the pineal gland and its energy affects the cerebrum.

ACTIVATING AND ENERGIZING THE CROWN CHAKRA

Do you often experience any of the following?

- Depression
- Tension
- Weak immune system
- Sleep disorder
- No spiritual awareness

- Chronic fatigue
- Chronic illness or mental disorder

If you face any of these, your crown chakra is clogged. There are various therapies that can help in activating it.

- Aroma therapy

Sage oil is the best remedy for negativity. Use it to ward off pessimism. You can also use jasmine, sandalwood, rosewood, or frankincense.

- Colour therapy

Place violet decorative candles in your house. White flowers like lilies, roses, and daisies can add beauty to your vases. Purple, gold, and white colour décor would add elegance to your home.

- Gemstone therapy

Amethyst and Quartz can stimulate this chakra. You can put a small piece of any of these stones under your pillow before sleeping.

- Nature therapy

Yoga in a park, or in a quiet place can really help. Meditation after a short nature walk will invigorate your senses.

- Sound therapy

Soothing, relaxing music can prove medicinal. Listen to music that you enjoy. It should work for you as a balm. You can also chant the mantra Om for it.

• Yoga therapy

You can try Sarvangasana and Matsyasana. For in-depth analysis refer to the chapter on Asanas.

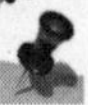

CROWN or SAHASRARA CHAKRA

Colour	Violet, white, gold
Associated Gland	Pineal
Principle	Purest being—the right to aspire
Location	Top of the head
Symbol	A 1000-petal lotus
Bodily Association	Cerebrum
Imbalances	Premature sexual maturity, headaches, photosensitivity, epilepsy, mental illness
Root Stimulants	Focusing on dreams. Violet foods like cabbage, pepper, brinjal and drinks, gemstones, clothing, and oils like jasmine and lavender

I hope this gives you a basic understanding of the marvel that is our body and what we can achieve if we understand the energy centres we possess. Since what I teach is a holistic approach to yoga, I feel it helps if you can understand how yoga can help release and enhance the flow of energy in our body. This is how it helps in dealing with certain health condition which I will talk about in Part Two of the book.

KRIYAS: PURIFICATION PROCESS

I often wonder how our lives have become the vanity box of toxins. As soon as you step out of the house, innumerable, invisible pollutants bump into you. Exposure to dust, pollen, germs, smoke, fungus, bacteria, chemicals, and viruses, has made all of us vulnerable to countless health issues. Like water needs to be purified of bacteria, our body too needs to be cleansed of unwanted impurities. But that can't happen on its own, can it? You need to detoxify your system regularly to be able to stay healthy and fit.

How long has it been since you actually felt good about yourself? Just stop for a moment and reflect on your life. Do you feel grumpy, irritable, or stressed? Are you suffering from allergies or health issues? Do you still fit into your old clothes? Are you too busy to even think or breathe right? Caught up in busy schedules, trying to fulfill responsibilities towards family and friends, have you completely forgotten yourself? Juggling between home and work, do you often feel the need to take a break and relax? If it is so, please stop neglecting yourself and your health. Take out time—be it an hour or only twenty minutes once in a few months and just detoxify. It is not asking too much, is it?

TRIDOSHAS

Have you ever wondered why all of us are so different? Your best friend might be restless while you may be calm and composed. Shreya might love parties, while Neha would love to sit back at home, read books and relax. Radhika might be extremely creative, while you may be very outgoing and adventurous. So what makes us unique? According to Ayurveda, there are three basic components that determine our individuality. Also known as Tridoshas, they are classified as:

1) Vata—Vata is the principle of development and change. It governs motion, breathing, circulation, and elimination, qualities that reflect the elements of space and air.
2) Pitta—It signifies transformation. Represented by digestion and metabolism, it governs our thoughts, experiences, emotions, and food habits, qualities that reflect the elements of fire and water.
3) Kapha—Kapha is the principle of protection, sustenance, and stability. It governs fluid balance and structure and helps build up muscle, fat, and bone, qualities that reflect the elements of water and earth.

WHAT'S YOUR DOSHA?

Derived from the five elements, doshas determine the blueprint of our personality. All of us have a certain amount of Vata, Pitta, and Kapha in our bodies. While all the three function together, by and large only one governs our constitution, and that is what influences our personality.

Do you want to find out what dosha is dominant in you? You need to balance it in order to maintain a healthy lifestyle. Take this quick, interesting quiz to find out. Before starting, be sure to mark the closest or most appropriate choice for best results.

1. Which of the following best describes your body structure?
A. Small, thin, lanky, or slender with prominent joints and weak muscles
B. Medium or well-proportioned with strong muscles
C. Large, heavy, broad, or stout

2. Your hair is:
A. Dry, brittle, wiry, or frizzy
B. Fine, thinning, soft, or prematurely grey
C. Abundant, thick, wavy or oily

3. How would you define your body weight?
A. Underweight
B. Average
C. Overweight or obese

4. Your skin is:
A. Rough, dull, or dry
B. Soft, oily, or prone to allergies
C. Thick, smooth, or pale

5. Your eyes are:
A. Small.
B. Sharp or penetrating
C. Big with thick lashes

6. Which of these define your appetite?
A. Small or irregular
B. Good, nutritious, or wholesome
C. Tendency of skipping meals

7. Your nails are:
A. Rough, dry, or brittle
B. Soft, pink and strong
C. Big or white

8. Which of the following best describes your sleep pattern?
A. Light, or easily awakened
B. Sound, moderate but less than 8 hours
C. Heavy, sound, excessive sleep

9. What can you say about your temperament?
A. Lively, restless and enthusiastic
B. Intense, expressive and motivated
C. Conservative and stubborn

10. What interests you the most?
A. Travel, art or philosophy
B. Sports and politics
C. Leisure activities

RESULT

Now that you have taken the quiz, total up your A's, B's, and C's and check your score. Your choice (maximum A's, B's or C's) determines the predominant dosha—one which needs balancing.

CHOICE: MOSTLY As RESULT: VATA DOSHA

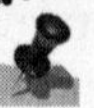

Characteristics of a Vata dominant person

Body Type	Thin, agile, narrow body structure
Skin Type	Dry, cool
Hair	Thin, dark, coarse, curly
Temperament	Creative, enthusiastic, short-tempered, restless, flexible
Libido	Sexually most active
Taste	Sour and salty

VATA

Vata literally means 'wind' or 'that which moves things'. It controls and gives motion to the other two doshas. Primarily located in the colon, joints, bones, thighs, skin, brain, and nerve tissues, this dosha triggers movement. Those governed by Vata are generally energetic, creative, flexible, and vivacious conversationalists. When there is an imbalance, the same people tend to become worrisome and often suffer from insomnia. Disciplined lifestyle, sound sleep, and regular eating habits are essential to maintain balance with people governed by Vata. Skipping meals, irregular digestion, and tension may lead not only to unintended weight loss but also unnecessary Vata imbalance.

Vata imbalance can be due to:

- Anxiousness, depression, stress
- Drinking alcohol, black tea, or coffee
- Smoking cigarettes

- Irregular eating and sleeping habits

There are several ways to balance your Vata. You can try:

- Meditation
- Light physical exercises—walking, yoga, swimming
- Sleeping early
- Eating at regular intervals

CHOICE: MOSTLY Bs RESULT: PITTA DOSHA

Characteristics of a Pitta dominant person

Body Type	Medium size and weight with muscular limbs and stable gait
Skin Type	Fair, soft, freckled, warm
Hair	Fine, soft, thinning, light with a tendency to grey soon
Temperament	Focused, intellectual, organized, witty, judgmental, articulate, proud
Libido	Moderately passionate
Taste	Sweet and bitter

PITTA

Pitta translates as 'that which cooks'. This dosha controls digestion, absorption, metabolism, and energy production. Primarily located in the small intestine, stomach, spleen, liver, blood, and pancreas it triggers transformation. Those governed by Pitta are sharp-witted, outspoken, courageous, and good decision makers. When imbalanced the same people tend to become egoistic, short-tempered, and argumentative. Nature walks, meditation, and regular daily routine are essential to maintain balance. Being overworked, excessively competitive and aggressive may lead to unnecessary Pitta imbalance.

Your Pitta can be imbalanced due to:

- Anger, rage, ego
- Drinking alcohol, black tea, or coffee
- Smoking cigarettes
- Work pressure

You can balance your Pitta with:

- Daily meditation
- Nature walks
- Balanced diet
- Avoiding artificial stimulants

CHOICE: MOSTLY Cs RESULT: KAPHA DOSHA

Characteristics of a Pitta dominant person

Body Type	Large, broad, well-developed frame with excellent stamina
Skin Type	Thick, oily, pale
Hair	Plentiful, thick, lustrous, wavy
Temperament	Calm, thoughtful, loving, compassionate, considerate
Libido	Strong, enduring sex drive
Taste	Sweet and spicy

KAPHA

Kapha simply means 'that which sticks'. It helps in the formation of fat, muscles, bones, and ligaments. Primarily located in the tissues, tendons, lungs, and lymph, it triggers protection. Those governed by Kapha are calm, selfless, loyal, affectionate, and supportive. If your Kapha is not balanced, you tend to become languid, dejected, and excessively overweight. Introspection, physical activity, and intellectual challenges are essential to maintain balance for people dominated by this dosha. Being a couch potato may lead to unnecessary Kapha imbalance.

Your Kapha can be imbalanced due to:

- Overeating
- Depression
- Being indoors
- Emotional disorder

To be able to bring balance to your Kapha, you can try:

- Writing
- Non-attachment
- Being assertive
- Wearing warm bright colours like red, orange, and yellow

KRIYAS—PURIFY YOURSELF

As I had said right at the beginning of the chapter, we need to cleanse ourselves regularly to enjoy our lives to the fullest. No amount of money can make you happy if you suffer from diseases and illnesses. Imbalanced tridoshas can lead to several health issues. To maintain equilibrium we need to detoxify our body. This can be done through kriyas.

In Sanskrit, the word kriya stands for 'action' or 'effort'. Kriyas are essentially yogic purification practices. Popularly known as Shatkarmas or 'six actions'; they aim at the holistic cleansing of our body, mind, and soul.

According to the traditional yoga, the six kriyas are as follows:

1. Neti—Nasal cleansing
2. Kapalabhati—Lungs cleansing through breathing
3. Trataka—Cleansing the mind through eyes
4. Dhauti—Cleansing the digestive tract
5. Nauli—Intestinal cleansing
6. Basti—Cleansing the colon
7. Shankhprakshalana—shorter version of cleansing the colon

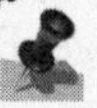

Before performing kriyas

Although kriyas are extremely beneficial in detoxifying the body, they must be done only under professional guidance. You should never try doing any of these kriyas on your own without the help of an expert.

10 benefits of kriyas

1. Help in overcoming countless diseases, they can be used as a form of yogic treatment.
2. Balance tridoshas and hence increase organizational skills.

3. Harmonize the body, mind, and soul.
4. Help in the free flow of our body's energy.
5. Stimulate good health and increases one's capacity to work.
6. Induce calmness of mind and create a heightened sense of awareness, concentration, and consciousness.
7. By converting negativity into positive energy, they help in releasing stress, apprehension, and tension.
8. Increase body's flexibility and facilitate the toning of external as well as internal organs.
9. Help in letting go of despair and pain.
10. Renew understanding of life and help in dismissing patterned thinking.

Now that we know the basics of kriyas, let us try and understand each of the 'six actions' in detail.

NETI KRIYA

Neti Kriya helps in cleaning the nasal tract through the nostrils. It effectively removes mucous and dirt from the nasal passage. For proper, regular breathing you need to keep your nostrils clean and germ-free. It is in fact a natural, safe and economical alternative to the many other nasal remedies available in the market.

BENEFITS OF NETI KRIYA

Regular practice of Neti Kriya can help combat various health issues like:

- Asthma
- Common cold
- Dust and pollen allergy
- Hay fever

- Headache
- Bad breath
- Dry or runny nose
- Inflammation or nose congestion
- Sinusitis
- Migraine
- Depression
- Tension

There are four types of Neti kriya depending upon the medium you use to perform it:

1. Jala Neti—with water
2. Dugdha Neti—with milk
3. Ghrita Neti—with ghee or clarified butter
4. Sutra Neti—with string

JALA NETI

The process of cleaning the nasal passage by salt water is known as Jala Neti. It is especially beneficial for those suffering from sinusitis, allergy, headache, or stress. A specially designed pot (Neti pot) is used for this purpose.

Priyanka, a 21-year-old aspiring model came to see me for chronic sinusitis. She lived in Pune and the damp weather there had deteriorated her condition. Under supervision, she tried Jala Neti Kriya and within a month her condition improved by 80 percent. Yes, it does work if performed correctly.

PROCEDURE

1. Fill your Neti Pot with warm salted water.
2. Slowly insert the pot's spout into one of your nostrils.

3. Bend forward, then tilt your head in such a way that the water flows out from the other nostril.

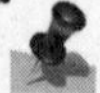

Tips for performing Jala Neti

While doing this kriya never breathe from your nose. No trace of water should remain in the nasal tract. Never rush the procedure. Take time to perform it correctly. Always practice Kapalabhati after Jala Neti. It will help in ejecting excessive water from your nose.

DUGDHA NETI

If you find salt water irritating, you can try Dugdha Neti. It is the process of cleansing the nasal passage through tepid, diluted milk poured into a neti pot. It is quite beneficial for those suffering from chronic nose bleeding.

PROCEDURE

1. Dilute milk with water and warm it to room temperature.
2. Pour it into a Neti pot and insert the spout into one nostril.
3 Tilt your head slightly so as to allow the milk to flow out of the other nostril.
4. Breathe through your mouth.

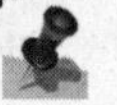

Tips for performing Dugdha Neti

Do not swallow the milk. If you experience any sort of pain, stop immediately and try and adjust the spout in such a way that the milk can flow freely. The milk should be free of any impurities. Also, pre-warm the milk and always use it at body temperature.

GHRITA NETI

Instead of water and milk you can also use warm ghee (clarified butter) to practice Ghrita Neti Kriya. If pure ghee is not available you can use unadulterated, chemical-free oil. Ghrita Neti is particularly beneficial in fighting against all diseases that manifest above the throat.

PROCEDURE

1. Use liquid ghee at body temperature.
2. Pour it into a Neti pot and insert the spout into one nostril.
3. Tilt your head slightly to allow the liquid ghee to flow out through the other nostril.

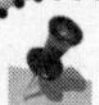

Tips for performing Ghrita Neti

Allow free passage of ghee from one nostril to the other. Practice near a basin. Do not continue if you feel suffocated. The ghee should be liquid, pure, and transparent.

SUTRA NETI

Sutra means thread and this neti is helpful when other conventional processes become ineffective due to minor nasal blockages. It is used to cure lethargy, hay fever, allergies, and excessive mucous. Do this kriya in the morning, after brushing your teeth. Use a 12 inch cotton thread dipped in beeswax for it.

PROCEDURE

1. Sit down and raise your neck a little.
2. Wet one end of the thread and insert it through one of your nostrils.

3. When the thread reaches your throat, very carefully and slowly take it out through your mouth.
4. Repeat the process with the other nostril as well.

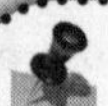

Tips for performing Sutra Neti

Unlike Jala Neti, Sutra Neti should be practiced only once or twice a week. Great care must be taken while administering the thread through your nasal passage. Take time to do this kriya. Do it only under supervision. Wash the thread properly after use.

KAPALABHATI

Kapalabhati is a yogic breathing technique used for the purification of the head and the lungs. It is practiced as pranayam as well as a kriya. It can help release not just stress, lethargy, and congestion but also volatile toxins from the body. It consists of successive, rapid, powerful exhalations followed by brief, passive inhalations. In Sanskrit kapala means 'skull' and bhati means 'to shine'. Thus Kapalabhati can be literally translated as a 'skull shining' or a 'skull cleaning' exercise. It gives prominence to exhalation, in quick spurts.

BENEFITS OF KAPALABHATI

I remember how my friend Renu was constantly worried about her 15-year-old son Sarthak preparing for his board examinations. Although Sarthak excelled at sports, she felt he could not focus on his studies. I advised her to try Kapalabhati, and after two months his grades improved. So who says yoga is only for older people? There are benefits in yoga for all age groups.

Regular practice of this kriya can help combat:

- Common cold
- Cough
- Sinusitis
- Bronchitis
- Tuberculosis
- Indigestion
- Gastritis
- Constipation
- Hyperacidity
- Obesity
- Asthma
- Blood impurities

Kapalabhati also:

- Increases concentration
- Improves digestion
- Increases heart rate and blood circulation
- Stimulates and regulates the glands
- Reduces stress, tension, and anxiety
- Cleanses nasal passages and respiratory system
- Helps treating diseases related to nervous system, endocrine system, circulatory system, and mental health

PROCEDURE

1. Sit comfortably in Padmasana or Siddhasana (refer to the chapter on Asanas for reference).
2. Rest your hands on your knees or lower belly.

3. Breathe normally for some time.
4 In a quick motion, contract your abdominal muscles and forcefully exhale all the air from your lungs.
5. Allow your lungs to fill without effort.
6. Perform this cycle ten times, allowing your breath to return to normal.
7. With regular practice you can increase the cycle to 120 times in each round.

Tips for doing Kapalabhati

You should practice Kapalabhati only on an empty stomach and increase the cycles gradually. Exhale quickly without giving heavy jerks. The number of rounds should be determined carefully. Do not continue if you feel dizzy or queasy. Keep your face muscles relaxed. Lastly, inhalation and exhalation should be uniform in all rounds.

WORD OF ADVICE

1. This kriya is not advisable for pregnant women.
2. Do not practice during the first three days of menstrual periods.
3. Not advisable for patients suffering from heart disease, high blood pressure, slip disc, and spondylosis.
4. Avoid doing it if you have fever, headache, abdomen pain, respiratory injury, or nose bleeding.
5. It should not be practised if you are suffering from any severe disease.

TRATAKA

College and school girls often ask me ways to increase attentiveness, memory, and sharpness. Competitiveness has increased anxiety and stress among students and most of them struggle to keep up. To boost concentration, Trataka comes across as an indispensable kriya. It is intended for developing mental alertness and involves constant, steady gazing at a particular spot or object without blinking. Also known as Yogic Gazing, it helps to get rid of unwanted thoughts and leads to the path of self-realization.

Basically Trataka is of two types:

a. Inner–In this the eyes remain closed while your attention is focused on the centre of your forehead.
b. Outer–Fixing eyes on some external object like candle, flame, sun, moon, or stars.

BENEFITS OF TRATAKA

This kriya helps combat:

- Mental disorders
- Negativity
- Eye disorders
- Instability
- Lack of concentration

EXERCISES

Trataka can be done in a lot of different ways. Choose the one which best suits you.

1. Close your eyes and focus all your attention on the middle of your forehead. Discontinue if you feel any kind of pain or discomfort. You might experience a slight tingling feeling.

2. On a white wall, draw a black dot and focus on it. If your walls are not white, you can hang a piece of white paper with a black dot on it.
3. Draw 'Om' on a piece of paper and gaze at it for two minutes.
4. Lie down on an open terrace and fix your eyes on the full moon or a particularly bright star.
5. Choose any source of light—candle or ghee-lamp and stare at the flame for a few minutes.
6. Look at a mirror and concentrate on the pupil of your eye.
7. At daybreak gaze at the sun for a few minutes. Do this exercise only under supervision.

PROCEDURE

1. Choose a quiet, secluded place to perform this kriya.
2. Sit on a mat in Siddhasana or Padmasana (see the chapter on Asanas for details). You can also lie down on a carpet.
3. In the beginning do it for two minutes only. Do not think about anything else. Concentrate only on the object or the centre of your forehead.
4. Gradually increase the time period.

Tips for doing Trataka

Do not tax your eyes by overdoing it. Sit quietly without fidgeting. If you want to try gazing at the sun, attempt it only under an expert guide. Do not let your mind wander while doing Trataka.

DHAUTI KRIYA

Detoxification is an important aspect of cleansing. I meet a lot of women who constantly complain of stomach disorders like acidity and constipation. Meera is 37 and has two beautiful school going children. She joined my yoga class a few months back and had a constant complaint of acidity. She wanted to try Dhauti Kriya to find relief. After doing it under the guidance of an expert, her digestion improved, and she feels happier and more energetic.

Changing food habits, unhealthy lifestyles, expanding waistlines, and fast food culture has made us susceptible to many diseases and health predicaments. Maintaining external hygiene is vital and that is why we take bath every day, isn't it? But why do we ignore the internal hygiene of our body which is equally important? For proper absorption, flushing out impurities within the body is indispensable. Dhauti Kriya—the process of cleaning the digestive tract and stomach is an important process of internal cleansing.

BENEFITS OF DHAUTI KRIYA

Dhauti Kriya helps combat:

- Asthma
- Diseases of spleen
- Cough and cold
- Constipation
- Gastritis
- Phlegm disorders
- Obesity

- Liver problems
- Bile disorders
- Diseases related to stomach
- Diabetes
- Eczema
- Tonsils
- Bad breath
- Arthritis

There are five different types of Dhauti Kriya:

a. Kunjal Kriya or Vaman Dhauti
b. Vastra Dhauti
c. Vatsara Dhauti
d. Agnisar Kriya

KUNJAL KRIYA

Vaman Dhauti or Kunjal Kriya cleanses the upper digestive tract and respiratory system. Like Jala Neti is used to clean the nasal tract, this kriya helps in cleaning the throat and stomach region. It is beneficial in the treatment of headache, constipation, gastric problems, indigestion, acidity, cough, cold, and asthma.

PROCEDURE

1. On an empty stomach drink four to eight glasses of lukewarm water mixed with a little salt. Drink the water as quickly as possible until you can't take in anymore.
2. Bend forward or sit on your heels and insert two fingers (middle and index) of your right hand into your mouth. Make sure that the fingers touch the back of your tongue.

3. Touch it till you feel like vomiting.
4. When you vomit bile and toxins too shall be ejected along with the saline water.
5. Repeat the procedure till all the water is ejected.

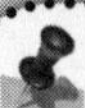

Tips for doing Kunjal Kriya

This kriya should be performed early in the morning on an empty stomach. Do it only once a week. Have a bowl of khichdi within an hour after practicing this kriya. If you are suffering from hyperacidity, use unsalted water. This kriya is not suitable for those suffering from high blood pressure, hernia, ulcers, cancer, and heart diseases.

VASTRA DHAUTI

It is a detoxification procedure used specifically to clean the stomach of mucous. A specially prepared cloth is used for this purification process. As it is a difficult kriya, it should not be practised without expert guidance.

PROCEDURE

1. Use a 2 inch broad and 20 feet long strip of clean muslin cloth. Dip it in lukewarm salty water.
2. Take one end of the cloth and slowly insert it in your mouth. Try swallowing it. Be very careful while performing this kriya.
3. If you are trying Dhauti kriya for the first time, try swallowing only one foot of the cloth. With practice you can increase the length.
4. Carefully draw out the cloth from your mouth.

Tips for doing Dhauti Kriya

This kriya should be practiced slowly. Do it only under expert guidance. It is best to do it on an empty stomach. Perform this kriya in a quiet and peaceful place.

VATSARA DHAUTI

Intestinal cleansing is a significant part of dhauti. Adequate supply of oxygen in the stomach is necessary for the proper functioning of our body. It is important to cleanse the body of impure, foul smelling gases. Vatsara Dhauti improves the digestive power of the body by enhancing the chemical reactions taking place within the stomach. It removes stale, unwanted gases and helps eliminate disorders like hyperacidity and heartburn.

PROCEDURE

1. Sit in a comfortable position.
2. Try creating vacuum in the stomach and inhale air.
3. Fill in the stomach as much as you can. Try gulping air if you find it difficult to perform it in one breath.
4. After your stomach has been filled in with air, relax comfortably for some time.
5. Do not exhale air. Allow it to come out on its own.

Tips for doing Vatsara Dhauti

You can practice this kriya once or twice, before eating. Do not try Vatsara Dhauti during or immediately after your meals.

AGNISAR KRIYA

I often meet women suffering from acute abdominal problems. Inadequate exercise, lack of proper movements, and deskbound lifestyle, causes lethargy. This affects the midriff causing kidney and liver related diseases, acidity, indigestion, and constipation. Priya, 42, I feel is a typical example. She works as a cashier in a bank and spends most of the day sitting at her desk. She doesn't exercise and recently she found out that her stomach ache was due to liver issues.

Agnisar Kriya is used to tighten and relax the abdominal muscles, giving the internal organs the much needed massage and exercise. Agni in Sanskrit stands for fire and therefore Agnisar is a practice which stimulates the body's inner fire and helps in its detoxification. It is an excellent remedy for digestive disorders like excessive gas, hyperacidity, heartburn, and stomach ache.

PROCEDURE

1. In a peaceful space, stand straight with a distance of 30 to 45 inches between your legs.
2. Place both hands on your thighs and keep your spine and arms erect.
3. Take a deep breath and exhale, contracting the abdomen and lungs so that all the air is expelled out.
4. While holding your breath in this position contract your abdominal muscles in and out. Do this rapidly without inhaling.
5. Repeat this procedure for as long as you can and then breathe slowly.

6. In the beginning you can start with 10 repetitions of contraction-expansion.
7. With practice you can increase it to 20–30 repetitions.

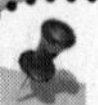

Tips for performing Agnisar Kriya

Perform this kriya early in the morning. Do not eat anything before performing it. Do it only after emptying the bowels. This kriya is not recommended if you are menstruating or pregnant. Do not practice if you are suffering from high BP, heart ailments, hyperthyroid, chronic diarrhea.

NAULI KRIYA

Nauli Kriya as you can guess by the name refers to naval cleansing. It is the process of eliminating accumulated impurities in the body. Increased mental and physical alertness helps you concentrate on work and at home. This kriya helps in regenerating, bracing, and energizing the alimentary system and the abdominal innards. Interestingly, this kriya also helps balance the body's Vata, Pitta, and Kapha. Some of its advantages include better breathing capacity, reduction in chronic constipation, toning of muscles, and strengthening of gastro-intestinal system.

BENEFITS OF NAULI KRIYA

This kriya helps combat:

- Constipation
- Nervousness
- Indigestion
- Acidity

- Flatulence
- Depression
- Hormonal imbalance
- Sexual and urinary disorders
- Diabetes
- Lethargy
- Emotional disturbances
- Diarrhea
- Lack of appetite
- Obesity

PROCEDURE

1. Stand straight with a distance of one foot between your legs.
2. Now bend and place your hands on your knees.
3. Exhale. Without inhaling perform Uddiyan Bandha (p. 169). Bend your neck so that it can touch your chin.
4. Transfer your body weight on the arms and relax your stomach.
5. Now squeeze in your abdominal region forcefully in circular motion.
6. With practice you can form the exact Nauli formation (tubular).

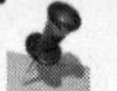

Tips for performing Nauli Kriya

Pregnant women should not try it. If you are planning to have a baby, even then you must avoid this kriya. Do not practice it during your menstruation cycle. Do not continue if you feel too exhausted. Practice this kriya only on an empty stomach. Never try it after your meals. Perform it in a standing position only. Also, you should do it only after your regular yoga session.

BASTI KRIYA

In Sanskrit, the word basti refers to the lower abdominal region—stomach, pelvis, and the bladder. It literally means enema and helps pass out accumulated faeces from the intestines. It is primarily used to cleanse the colon through the rectum. Water is first sucked into the large intestine through the anus and then thrown out. Since this kriya quite difficult, only advanced yoga practitioners should perform it. Nonetheless, with practice you can learn how to do it but medical advice and doctor's approval is necessary before performing it.

BENEFITS OF BASTI KRIYA

Regular practice can help combat:

- Dropsy
- Bile and phlegm related diseases
- Urinary disorders
- Indigestion
- Constipation
- Depression
- Hormonal imbalance
- Sexual and urinary disorders
- Diabetes
- Lethargy
- Emotional disturbances
- Diarrhea
- Lack of appetite
- Obesity
- Blood purification

There are two types of Basti Kriya:

a. Sthala Basti
b. Jala Basti

STHALA BASTI

Sthala in Sanskrit means ground. This kriya cleanses the colon by sucking in air through the anus, without the help of any external aid. It is performed on ground unlike Jala Basti which is practiced using water. Acidity and gas problems can be easily resolved through this process.

PROCEDURE

1. Lie on your back and bend your knees towards your chest.
2. Now slowly raise your buttocks and contract your anal muscles so as to suck in the air.
3. Move the air in and take it out as flatulence.

Tips for performing Sthala Basti

Do not practice this kriya if you are suffering from high blood pressure, digestive disorders, or hernia. This should be performed on an empty stomach. It must be performed without clothes.

JALA BASTI

Jala stands for water and this kriya cleanses the colon by sucking water into the anus. It is more effective than Sthala Basti and also helps in combating foul mouth odour, skin problems, obesity, and depression. Jala Basti helps create positivity around you, slowing down your mood swings and invigorating your sexual desires.

PROCEDURE

1. Use a 13-15 inch long hollow bamboo or plastic tube. Lubricate it well with beeswax or Vaseline.
2. Slowly insert 4 inches of the tube into your anus and sit over a basin of water in Utkatasana (see p. 174).
3. Exhale. Try sucking in the water through the anus with the help of the tube.
4. Perform this kriya until you can hold it no longer. Then remove the tube without exhaling.
5. Stand up and exhale slowly through the nose.
6. Now squat over the toilet so that the water can come out.
7. With practice you'll be able to perform this kriya without the catheter.

Tips for performing Jala Basti

Perform it on an empty stomach. The tube must be sterilized before and after use. The water should be neither too cold nor hot. Use lukewarm water in winters. Make sure that all the water is expelled. Do not try it during monsoons since this kriya generates heat in the body.

SHANKHAPRAKSHALANA

Shankhaprakshalana is made up of two words—'Shankh' meaning conch and 'Prakshalana' which refers to cleaning thoroughly. Conch represents the entire alimentary canal that is cleansed by practising this Kriya.

PROCEDURE

1. Boil 3 quarts of water and let it cool.
2. Then add sea salt or Himalayan salt. Do not use refined common salt and additives (a teaspoon per litre).
3. Drink two glasses of lukewarm saltwater.
4. Perform the four movements in 'Cycle of Movements'.
5. Drink two glasses of lukewarm water.
6. Perform the four-stroke cycle again.
7. Continue like this until you have drunk six glasses. This is a full water intake cycle.
8. Go to the bathroom and wait for evacuation to occur. If not produced within five minutes, repeat the cycle of movements, without water.
9. The four postures are: 1) Tadasana 2) Trikonasana 3) Vakrasana 4) Bhujangasana

Tips for performing Shankhaprakshalana

You should perform Shankhaprakshalana only under the supervision of an expert and once or twice a year during the change of season. After performing this Kriya, a whole day of rest is recommended. Your teacher can guide you on what to eat and when after you perform this cleansing process. People who suffer from ulcers, heart disease, blood pressure, epilepsy or kidney ailments should not do Shankhaprakshalana except under medical supervision.

With this I hope you will have the basic understanding about kriyas and why these cleansing methods are useful for us. We clean our clothes, homes, even our external bodies. So why not the insides of our bodies? Try these under the guidance of an expert and experience the difference in your well-being.

PRANAYAM: BREATHE IN, BREATHE OUT

Breath is the essence of our existence. Our life and health is connected to our breathing intrinsically. But do we actually pay attention to our breathing? We can live without food or water for days, but without breathing we would surely die. Why is it so? Proper breathing performs two vital functions: it brings much needed oxygen to the bloodstream and controls prana—the universal life force. Pranayam is the science of breath control through successive exercises that help in maintaining overall health. It is beneficial in energizing our bodies and providing the fuel for our existence.

THE FOUR STAGES OF BREATHING

Proper breathing utilizes the power of our lungs. Thousands of years ago, yogis realized the importance of adequate oxygen supply. They developed and perfected various breathing techniques over the ages. This helped later generations to revitalize the mind and invigorate the body.

Breathing channelizes energy to our body through four stages—inhalation, internal retention, exhalation, and external retention. The ratio between these stages should ideally be 1:4:2:4. Did you know that exhalation is one of the most significant part of breathing? Yes, its true. It helps to remove carbon dioxide and other impurities from our body. With regular and proper practice of Pranayam, you can not only improve your immune system but also become stress free. It trains you to use your lungs to the maximum capacity so that the cells in the body are oxygenated well.

To understand Pranayam you need to first understand the four basic stages of breathing.

1. Puraka or inhalation

The first stage of breathing is known as Puraka or inhalation. While practicing Pranayam, your inhalation should be slow and controlled. In yogic terms, one single inhalation is known as Puraka. This stage helps you draw in air smoothly and uniformly. Since it is a continuous process, you should inhale without any kind of interruption.

2. Abhyantara kumbhaka or internal retention

Abhyantara Kumbhaka is performed right after Puraka. During this stage you intentionally stop the flow of air and hold it in your lungs, without any internal or external movement. In the beginning you might experience some discomfort and may also have to use force to remain still. But eventually, with practice you can master this stage to stay calm and focused.

3. Rechaka or exhalation

Rechaka is the third stage performed right after Abhyantara Kumbhaka. Even though the pace may differ, the exhaled air should be released uniformly and continuously like the first stage. Unlike inhalation, exhalation involves the relaxation of tensed muscles.

4. Bahya kumbhaka or external retention

The last stage of breathing is known as Bahya Kumbhaka. During this stage you intentionally pause after exhalation. This break is intentional and is done right before starting a new cycle of breathing.

THE IMPORTANCE OF HEALTHY BREATHING

Breathing is spontaneous and occurs naturally to everyone. Yet most of us do not know how to breathe correctly. In this chapter I want to focus on the essentials of breathing and how Pranayam plays an important role in it.

Do you often experience shortness of breath? This can be caused due to various reasons. Slouching and bad posture reduce our lung capacity and hamper our breathing. Moreover, sedentary lifestyle, demanding jobs, tension, and fatigue lead to decreased levels of blood circulation. Shallow breathing reduces vitality and makes us vulnerable to various diseases. It can cause insomnia, fatigue, muscle cramps, flatulence, dizziness, heartburn, visual impairment, chest congestion, weak immune system, nervousness, stomach problems, and mental disorders.

A large chunk of our need for energy is fulfilled by the air we breathe. Oxygen is the most important nutrient in the body, essential for the proper functioning of the brain, nerves, glands, and all other internal organs. It recharges and purifies the bloodstream. This in turn boosts every part of the body making it youthful and animated. Lack of oxygen can cause numerous health problems including cancer, stroke and heart attack. **Good health is directly proportional to proper breathing.** It is the only process which supplies oxygen to various organs and helps in cleansing the body of waste products and toxins.

WHAT IS PRANAYAM?

The word Pranayam is derived from two words, prana and ayam. Prana stands for essential energy or consciousness which is present in each one of us. In simple terms it may be understood as breath. Ayam on the other hand, stands for stretching or expansion. It is the fourth limb of Ashtanga yoga and is also known as the 'Heart of Yoga'. It is the science of breath regulation and control which consists of a series of exercises intended to meet our physical and mental needs.

Once you understand how to balance, relax, and expand the breath, the respiratory system is fortified, nervous system is relieved, and the body is well oxygenated. Following a rhythmic pattern of slow and deep breathing can help in relaxing the body. You reach a state of profuse liveliness, peaceful vibrancy, and pleasant well-being. This is what I would term as a precursor to good health and can effectively and can effectively prevent major diseases and cure minor ailments.

BENEFITS OF PRANAYAM

Pranayam has a holistic effect on the mind and body. It supervises not only the physical body and the mind but also helps in the realization of the self. It is the best method to bust anxiety and can also work as a superb spiritual energizer. Once you start practicing it, you'll observe changes in your body. It will become strong, vibrant, and healthy. All psychological dilemmas, nervousness, stress, qualms, and doubts will start diminishing. Pranayam is indeed a storehouse of miraculous benefits; some of which include:

a. Calming the nerves
b. Improving the functioning of the heart
c. Reducing extra fat
d. Improving digestion
e. More resilience to diseases
f. Combating lethargy and fatigue
g. Increasing concentration power
h. Breathing becoming more regular
i. Dealing with mental conditions like depression, negativity, stress, and anxiety
j. Improving our quality of life
k. Helping combat back ache, rheumatism, stiff joints, and muscle sprain
l. Revitalizing lost endurance
m. Preparing the mind for meditation
n. Inducing lightness of body, inner peace, better sleep, and sharp memory
o. Helping combat problems like obesity, acidity, cancer, insomnia, low blood pressure, migraine, respiratory disorders, depression, sinusitis, flatulence, asthma, skin ailments, allergy, heart diseases, lung congestion, high blood pressure, sexual infirmities, kidney problems, constipation, diabetes, and high cholesterol

BEFORE YOU BEGIN

Before you begin practicing Pranayam, you need to know a few important things.

THINGS TO KEEP IN MIND

Clothes	Light, comfortable clothes. Should not be tight around the waist.
Food intake	Should not be tried immediately after meals. Practice on an empty stomach. You can however do it 4 hours after a meal. Eat light, fresh food.
Location	Open spaces are best for Pranayam. However you can try it at home. If you practice it in a room, it should be well ventilated.
Posture	The back of your neck should be aligned with your spinal cord. You must not slouch. Keep your back and spine comfortably erect.
Medical condition	Do not practice any of the advanced exercises if you are sick. However you can practice Pranayam for beginners.
Effort required	Never strain yourself while practising Pranayam. Any kind of stress on your body or muscles means you should stop immediately.
Precautions	Practice in a cool, calm place.

PRANAYAM FOR BEGINNERS

Now that you know what Pranayam is, allow me tell you some of its basic techniques which can be practised by anyone and everyone. If you have a busy schedule and hardly find time to exercise, you can try these out. The exercises form the backbone of pranayam and should be practiced before your daily set of asanas. They have numerous health benefits, are easy to follow, and do not require any kind of extra effort. Let us understand each one in detail.

ANULOM VILOM

Anulom Vilom, also known as alternate nostril breathing, is an excellent Pranayam which helps bust stress and anxiety. By purifying the mind as well as the body, it improves our overall health. In this Pranayam we inhale through one nostril, retain the breath, and exhale through the other nostril. It is one of the most popular Pranayams and you must have seen it being performed on TV in yoga camps or sessions. Interestingly, it can be practiced by people of all age groups. As opposed to Kapalabhati, in this technique, you use the lungs for breathing instead of the abdomen.

Procedure

a. Close your eyes and sit in a relaxed position.
b. Close your right nostril with your right thumb and exhale from your left nostril. The exhalation should be deep and slow.
c. Now inhale slowly from the left nostril and then close it with your ring finger. Simultaneously open your right nostril and exhale. Now inhale from the right nostril, close it and exhale from the left nostril.
d. This completes one cycle. In the beginning you can repeat the procedure 10 cycles. Gradually increase the repetitions to 50.

Benefits

a. Anulom Vilom increases the oxygen intake and reduces stress and anxiety. It makes you feel calm and peaceful.
b. It can cure hypertension, high blood pressure, diabetes, obesity, cancer, migraine, heart problems, snoring, acidity, paralysis, and asthma.
c. Dispels negativity and helps you approach everything with a positive outlook.
d. Can help combat sexual and reproductive disorders.
e. Problems related to urinary tract, eyes, and nose can also be resolved.

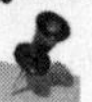

Tips for performing Anulom Vilom

- Breathe only through your lungs. Do not breathe through your stomach.
- Practice slowly. Your breathing should be rhythmic.
- Sit in a relaxed position. Do not try Anulom Vilom if you are stressed out.
- Discontinue if you feel wobbly or lightheaded.

CHANDRABHEDAN

Chandrabhedan is derived from the words 'chandra' and 'bheda'. Chandra stands for the moon and bheda means to pass through. It calms the body and relaxes the mind. In this pranayam you inhale through the left nostril in order to invigorate the other organs. The left nostril represents lunar energy and hence the name.

Procedure

a. Sit in a meditative pose or in a comfortable position on the floor.
b. Keep your shoulders and back relaxed.
c. Now close your right nostril with your right hand thumb.
d. Inhale from the left nostril.
e. Close the left nostril with the right hand's index and middle fingers.
f. Now exhale from the right nostril.
g. Gradually increase the number of rounds to 20.

Benefits

a. It cools the body by reducing the flow of bile.
b. It is also useful for meditation.
c. Skin diseases can be cured by this Pranayam.
d. It also steadies the mind and induces muscular relaxation.
e. It reduces stress, hypertension by relaxing the nervous system.
f. It is beneficial against heartburn and laziness.

Tips for performing Chandrabhedan

- Avoid it if you suffer from low blood pressure.
- People suffering from asthma, cough and cold, and constipation should not try it.
- Do not perform more than 20-25 rounds.
- Do not perform Chandrabhedan and Suryabhedan on the same day.
- This technique should be tried only during summers. Do not practice it in winters.

SURYABHEDAN

Surya stand for sun and bhedan means to pierce. In Suryabhedan Pranayam one inhales through the right nostril, the seat of solar energy. It is especially good for people suffering from depression, lethargy, and dullness.

Procedure

a. Sit comfortably in a meditative posture.
b. Close your left nostril with the index and middle finger of the right hand.
c. Inhale from your right nostril.
d. Now close the right nostril with your right hand thumb.
e. Exhale through the left nostril.
f. Repeat the cycle. You can gradually try practising 20 rounds.

Benefits

a. It generates body heat and hence increases energy levels.
b. The brain gets stimulated and the immune system becomes stronger.
c. Helps women suffering from sexual disorders. Increases libido.
d. Digestion is improved and problems of flatulence and acidity are reduced.
e. Helps to purify blood and frees the body of impurities.
f. It can also help in stimulating the chakras.
g. Induces longevity.

Tips for performing Suryabhedan

- People suffering from heart problems, acidity, and hypertension should not try it.
- This pranayam should be performed only during winters.
- Do not perform it if you are suffering from fever. This Pranayam increases body heat.

While practising the above basic Pranayams soften your facial muscles and let your entire body be deeply relaxed. You must always be at ease and breathe comfortably. Pranayam is an extremely gentle and subtle technique. If you ever feel any sort of uneasiness, anxiety, or strain, stop immediately and rest for a while. Take your time, and feel each breath.

ADVANCED PRANAYAM

Now that you have kick started your basic breathing routine, let us try and understand a few other important techniques. In the Vedas, 50 different breathing exercises have been mentioned. Not all are important for your understanding. I will focus on some other significant Pranayams that can be tried by advanced practitioners. You should perform these only under the guidance of an expert.

BHRAMARI

Derived from the word 'bhramar' or humming bee, Bhramari Pranayam is considered as the best breathing exercise for meditation. While performing it one produces the sound of a humming bee and hence it is also known as bee breath. It not only relaxes the brain but also reduces mental stress, fatigue, and high blood pressure. This technique can be tried by anyone—children, old people, and pregnant women can also try it. It instantly calms down the mind and relieves it of tension, anger, frustration, and anxiety.

Procedure

a. Sit in a quiet, airy place in any comfortable asana with your eyes closed. The surrounding should be peaceful and you should feel calm while performing this Pranayam.
b. Use both your hands in this step. Close your ear with the thumb and let your forefinger rest on the forehead. The other three fingers should be placed in such a way that they cover your eyes and rest right above the base of your nose.
c. Now inhale deeply and make a high-pitched sound while exhaling out. It should be similar to the buzz of a humming bee.
d. Continue the same procedure 5–10 times.
e. After the Pranayam stay quiet for a few minutes. Observe the stillness around you and the calmness within.
f. You can try it 3 to 4 times a day.

Benefits

a. It is helpful for people suffering from depression, hypertension, blood pressure, paralysis, migraine, and headache.
b. Reduces anger and improves concentration and memory.
c. Helps build confidence and relieves all sorts of tension.
d. It is the best meditative Pranayam. It can also awaken the chakras.
e. By regulating the endocrine system it can also be helpful during pregnancy. It facilitates easy and hassle free delivery.

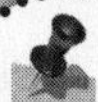

Tips for performing Bhramari

- Never insert your finger inside your ear while doing this Pranayam.
- Do not press your fingers. It should rest comfortably on your forehead, eyes and ears.
- Perform this technique only on an empty stomach. Do it atleast four hours after your last meal.
- While making the humming sound, make sure that your mouth is closed.

BHASTIRIKA

A combination of Kapalabhati and Anulom Vilom, Bhastirika in Sanskrit stands for bellows. It involves deep inhalation and exhalation so that the body gets the maximum amount of oxygen. Forceful exhalation is the most important step in this Pranayam. It not only improves metabolism and helps you lose weight but also improves your resistance power and helps keep diseases at bay.

Procedure

a. Sit on the floor in a meditative pose or in any comfortable position.
b. Keep your back straight and your shoulder muscles relaxed.
c. Do kapalabhati 25 times, holding the last stroke while breathing out. Then do 1 set of Anulom Vilom. This forms one round of Bhastirika Pranayam.

Benefits

a. It helps release toxins.
b. By increasing the body heat it opens up the body's energy pathways.
c. Naturally reduces extra fat and helps against obesity and laziness.
d. It enhances digestion.
e. Relieves throat inflammation.
f. Regulates and fortifies the nervous system.
h. Boosts oxygen supply and helps in blood purification.

Tips for performing Bhastirika

- Avoid this Pranayam if you suffer from high blood pressure, heart diseases, tuberculosis, asthma, lung problems, hernia, or hypertension.
- Pregnant women should avoid it.
- Do not practice this if you are feeling physically unfit.
- Do it only once a day for 3-5 minutes.
- Avoid performing it during summers.

KAPALABHATI

Also known as forceful exhalations, the word kapalabhati is derived from the words kapala and bhati. Kapala means skull and bhati means light. An extremely stimulating abdominal breathing exercise, it involves natural inhalation followed by forceful exhalation. The technique is used for releasing bodily toxins and cleansing it of impurities. The breath is quick, short, and forceful.

Procedure

a. Sit in a comfortable position in an open area or a well ventilated room. Your mind should be at peace and face should be relaxed. Do not try Kapalabhati under any kind of stress.
b. Inhale twice. Your breathing should be deep and through both the nostrils. While inhaling your abdomen should inflate. Now gently exhale all the air from your lungs. While exhaling, you should forcefully contract your abdominal muscles.
c. Exhale quickly with your mouth closed. The sound should be like a gentle sneeze
d. Your focus should be on your lower belly. The belly should contract and expand as you inhale and exhale.
e. Now inhale and exhale in quick rhythmic succession
f. Your inhalation and exhalation should be quick. Use only your abdominal area for breathing.
g. Perform 20-25 cycles in the beginning. You can gradually increase the repetition to 100 cycles.

Benefits

a. It cleanses the lungs and respiratory system. It keeps at bay diseases like common cold, cough, sinusitis, tuberculosis, and bronchitis.
b. Improves digestion and absorption. It helps in combating indigestion, constipation, flatulence, acidity, and gastric problems.

c. Strengthens the nervous system and helps in the functioning of the circulatory system.
d. Helps fight obesity and reduces abdominal fat deposits.
e. Energizes the mind and prepares it for meditation.
f. Purifies blood and the supply of oxygen to body cells also increases.

Tips for performing Kapalabhati

- Do not repeat if you feel any kind of discomfort, pain, or dizziness
- Never contract your abdomen while inhaling
- Do not practice during menstruation or if you are pregnant
- Quick breathing should not be from the chest but only from the abdominal area
- Never practice Kapalabhati right after meals. It should always be done on an empty stomach
- Your shoulders and back should not move during the exercise
- Do not practice if you are suffering from hernia, heart problems, blood pressure, spondylosis, or asthma
- Exhalation should be forceful but comfortable. Do not pressurize your body

SHEETKARI

Sheet means 'cool' and hence Sheetkari means 'that which cools'. Also known as teeth hissing Pranayam, it has a cooling effect on the body and the mind. The nerve channels are energized and you will feel at peace through this Pranayam.

It also controls acidity and stomach disorders, thirst, hunger and brings down the body temperature.

Procedure

a. Sit on the floor in a comfortable position.
b. Keep your back and shoulders relaxed.
c. Place your hands on the knees. Keep your fingers relaxed and your eyes closed.
d. Join your upper and lower teeth.
e. Fix the front portion of your tongue against the front teeth and the rest of the tongue on the palate.
f. Separate your lips and inhale from the mouth making a chilling sound.
g. Retain your breath for as long as possible.
h. Now exhale through both nostrils.
i. This completes one round of Sheetkari Pranayam.

Benefits

a. Interestingly, this Pranayam helps in curing all sorts of dental diseases.
b. It brings down the body temperature.
c. Your body complexion will become clearer.
d. It helps control high blood pressure.
e. It also purifies your blood.
f. Helps combat indigestion, fever, and acidity.
g. Try this Pranayam to keep your teeth and gums healthy.

Tips for performing Sheetkari

- Do not try this if you have low blood pressure.
- It is not recommended for people suffering from high fever, cold, cough, asthma, sinusitis, or bronchitis.
- Do not practice it if you are suffering from heart diseases.
- Should be avoided in winters.

SHEETALI

It is a breathing technique similar to Sheetkari Pranayam. Sheetal means calmness. It brings down the body temperature and hence is also known as the cooling breath technique. Sheetali uses the tongue to cool down the body and the mind.

Procedure

a. Sit in a comfortable position.
b. Close your eyes and relax your body. Breathe normally.
c. Put your tongue on the lower lip and try rolling it.
d. Inhale deeply from the mouth.
e. Retain your breath for as long as possible.
f. Now slowly close your mouth and exhale through your nose.
g. In the beginning try 2-3 rounds. Gradually increase it up to 15 rounds.

Benefits

a. It cools the body as I had mentioned.
b. Toxins are reduced by doing it as it cleanses the blood.
c. Tumor, fever, indigestion, constipation, jaundice, skin disorders can also be combated through it.

d. It cures acidity and hypertension.
e. It is good for people who have anger issues. It makes the body calm and reduces tension.
f. It also relieves indigestion and bile disorders.
g. Eyes and skin disorders can also be treated.
h. If you are suffering from tonsils this Pranayam can be really helpful.

Tips for performing Sheetali Pranayam

- Do not try it in winters.
- Avoid this Pranayam if you are suffering from cough and cold.
- Not recommended for people suffering from asthma, bronchitis or tuberculosis.
- Avoid it if you are suffering from chronic constipation.

UJJAYI

Also known as ocean breath, this Pranayam concentrates, directs, and warms the breath before it enters the lungs. In this technique one breathes through the throat instead of the nose. It stimulates the metabolic rate by increasing the blood circulation. It also helps the lungs to absorb more oxygen and improves concentration.

Procedure

a. Sit straight in a comfortable position.
b. Inhale slowly and deeply through both your nostrils.
c. Try holding your breath. Do it for as long as possible.
d. Now exhale slowly with a whispering sound. While doing this step, contract your air passage.

e. Begin by doing 2-3 rounds. You can gradually increase it to 20 rounds.

Benefits

a. Ujjayi Pranayam stimulates the thyroid glands to balance the hormones in the body.
b. The respiratory and nervous systems work better if one practises this Pranayam.
c. It strengthens the vocal cords.
d. Disorders related to the digestive system can also be reduced.
e. It stimulates the thyroid gland.
f. It improves blood circulation and fights against lung diseases like tuberculosis and asthma.
g. Diseases related to the chest and the throat can also be combated.

Tips for performing Ujjayi

- Begin by doing this pranayam for 3-5 minutes. You can gradually increase the time period to 15 minutes.
- People suffering from heart diseases should not try this.
- The ratio of inhalation and exhalation should be 1:2.

Our breath is what is constant throughout our lives. Our breathing gets altered with our moods, physical activity and sometimes due to the hormones. It is also one of the most important component of all yoga exercises. When we get down to the workouts in Part Two, a basic understanding about breathing will help you achieve perfection in doing asanas and bring you the maximum benefits.

ASANAS: TRANSFORM YOURSELF

Look around you. Do you often come across people engrossed on their smart phones or busy chatting online? I recently read a disturbing news item about how a teenager in Mumbai lost his life in a road accident while listening to music. Communication and social media has become a part of our daily lives, yet most of us are victims of loneliness. We feel left out with often not too many 'real' people to talk to. In the virtual world of floating identities, life has transformed into a series of unaccomplished realities. We pretend to be what we are not, trying hard to climb the ladder of fame and ambition. In the long run, what we fail to understand is that we aren't doing justice to ourselves or our bodies. In such a situation coping with stress, anxiety, tension, depression, and loneliness becomes all the more difficult.

What can we do to make our lives better? Look and feel calm and happy? You won't be surprised to know that yoga, one of the oldest sciences of life can be beneficial in healing our modern day anxieties. Yoga can help you slow down, relax, and heal physically, mentally, as well as spiritually. In fact, the best part is that anyone can learn asanas. No matter how old you are, how much you weigh, you can easily practise yoga. Asanas are not theoretical but a practical way of life. They not only help tone the external parts of your body but also nurse the internal organs. Moreover, you do not even require special clothes or equipment to do it. All you need is some space, a little will power, and a strong desire to lead a healthier life.

Why should I try asanas? How long will I have to do it? What are its long term benefits? Will it work for me? What if it doesn't? I am sure many such questions have popped up in your mind. All I'd like to say is that; don't jump to conclusions before you begin. Try it once and you will yourself understand the miraculous effects of yoga.

TESTING YOUR YOGA IQ

Yoga and asanas are quite in vogue nowadays. But do you really understand its meaning and significance? Let's find out through this interesting quiz.

1. What does the word yoga mean?
a. The union of all living and non-living objects
b. The union of mind, body, and soul
c. The union of mind, body, and spirit in communication and consciousness
d. The union of sun, moon, and stars

2. How old is the yogic system?
a. 200 years
b. 5000 years
c. 50 years
d. 2000 years

3. Yoga asanas are designed for:
a. Improving fitness
b. Creating a balance between the mind, body, and soul

c. Enhancing awareness
d. All of the above

4. How many poses make up one sun salutation?
a. 12
b. 14
c. 10
d. 16

5. Which type of postures should you try if you are menstruating?
a. Twisting postures
b. Light back bending
c. Forward bends
d. Deep back bending

6. Which of the following asanas can be tried during pregnancy?
a. Trikonasana
b. Sukhasana
c. Shavasana
d. All of the above

7. The most relaxing yoga pose is?
a. Shavasana
b. Tadasana
c. Padmasana
d. Chakrasana

8. When buying a yoga mat, the most important thing to be kept in mind is:
a. Price
b. Shape

c. Stability
d. Colour

9. Suryanamaskar is the favourite asana of:
a. Neha Dhupia
b. Bipashan Basu
c. Aishwarya Rai
d. Kareena Kapoor

10. Pranayama is:
a. Breath control
b. Meditation
c. Relaxation
d. A kriya

To find out the answers refer to page 118 at the end of this chapter.

UNDERSTANDING YOGA

Now that you know the basics, let us try and understand yoga a little better.

Yoga derives its roots from India, where it originated thousands of years ago. It is, in fact, the world's oldest system of individual advancement and embraces the body, mind, as well as the spirit. Developed over many eons, yoga is an evolving science that continues to grow, rendering to our various needs.

A lot of young girls I know want to try yoga for flexible limbs and overall fitness so that they can look great and feel good about their body. Women come to me seeking relief from ailments like stress, queasiness, backache or weight issues.

Whatever be the problem, I feel yoga offers the best solutions. It can be practised by everyone, irrespective of their gender, age, or body type. It is also all encompassing and by increasing your overall awareness, yoga can bring a subtle transformation in the way you perceive life. Creating a protective layer of inner peace, yoga has the power to envelope you in a state where the mind is calm and the body is stress-free and relaxed. With minimal side effects, it is an exceptional curative for most diseases.

Based on different approaches to life, yoga can be divided into four paths. Interestingly, the final purpose of each path is the same—coming together with the Divine Being or God. The four paths are as follows:

1. Karma Yoga—Karma is the Sanskrit term for deed or action, hence this path is also known as the yoga of action. It is suitable for extroverts and outgoing people and its main objective is to purify the heart by teaching altruism. Selfless service helps in dispelling ego and therefore teaches discipline. Through Karma Yoga, you can easily eliminate the feelings of hatred, covetousness, insensitivity, gluttony, and selfishness. This path of yoga changes your perception and the way you look at life.
2. Bhakti Yoga—Also known as devotional yoga, it is the path of piety that predominantly appeals to sensitive, emotional people. It is stimulated by love and perceives God as its embodiment. Chants and devotional songs are an essential part of Bhakti Yoga. It banishes the feelings of abhorrence,

possessiveness, vanity, egotism, and haughtiness. It infuses the feelings of happiness, pleasure, divine joy, harmony, amity, and knowledge. It is among the easiest of all the paths since it does not depend upon human tendencies.

3. Jnana Yoga—It is the multidimensional path of awareness and wisdom. Considered to be the most difficult, it requires great will power and intelligence. One uses the mind to investigate its innate nature. Self-realization of the Supreme Self is necessary for a person who wants to be independent from the bonds of life. Jnana Yoga is however not meant for the general masses. A great deal of knowledge and practice is required so as to follow and understand this challenging path. Meditation is integral to it and requires a lot of patience and strong will. A person who follows it attains tranquility, fortitude, abstinence, and self-control.
4. Ashtanga Yoga—It literally means the King of Yoga. It is the path which deals in the science of physical and mental control. It not just turns the mental and physical energy into spiritual energy but also helps one perceive life as an insider. In Ashtanga Yoga, the mind is used as an instrument to look into the depths of one self. Such perception not only brings about self-realization but also leads to divinity. These appendages are in fact an advancing series of steps leading to enlightenment through the cleansing of the body and the mind.

ASANAS DECODED

Now that you know that asanas are a part of Ashtanga Yoga, let us try and understand its meaning. What are asanas? Asana is the Sanskrit term for 'body posture'. Hundreds of distinctive asanas form the core of yoga. Designed to promote good health and a state of mental and physical well being, these postures help in the proper functioning of the body by balancing the mind. Asanas not only help in stretching, but also help in opening the energy channels, chakras, and cognitive centres of the body. Endowed with healing properties, these simple postures can help you in rejuvenating and enlivening your mind, body, and soul. Asanas have a lot of benefits.

1. It promotes all-round fitness. Holistic health is possible through asanas.
2. You can lose weight by practising asanas like Suryanamaskar (p. 119) and Kapalabhati (p. 98).
3. It improves the elasticity of the body, making it agile and flexible.
4. It strengthens the muscles and ligaments, making them resilient.
5. Regular practice helps improve the overall balance of the body, improving the posture of your body.
6. A great stress buster, asanas can help combat depression, anxiety, and tension.
7. Many diseases like hypertension, constipation, excessive fat, diabetes, asthma, and acidity can be cured.
8. Can also be beneficial during pregnancy and menstruation.
9. Detoxification is one of the most vital constituents of asanas.
10. Body ache, back pain, joint pain, and headache are also reduced.
11. By relaxing the mind and body, it can also help you in having better relationships with people around you.

Mental satisfaction, happiness, and peace are some of the most important benefits of asanas.

12. You can also live longer and better if you incorporate asanas in your daily routine.
13. Immunity can also be improved through regular practice of asanas. Pranayam and other breathing exercises help build up stamina.
15. Asanas can also help you sleep better.

ASANAS FOR EVERYONE

Asanas are easy to follow and can be done by everyone. It does not matter how old or young you are or if you have never exercised in your life. You can also start at the beginners' level under the guidance of an expert and then progress gradually to the next level depending on your fitness. My dad is in his sixties and he begins his day with a session of yoga. He feels energized and rejuvenated, and hates to miss a single session.

I met Riya the other day. She is 16-years-old and had a problem of irregular periods. Pari, 19, loves ice cream but feels scared to have it because of her tonsillitis. And newly married Ritu cannot go to Manali for her honeymoon. The reason is simple. She has asthma and her condition worsens in hilly areas. Every one of you know how irritating and problematic such ailments can be. Don't you want to get rid of such problems and lead a better, healthier life? Asanas can surely help you in attaining good health. I have created a list of asanas for specific diseases and health problems so that you can combat them with ease. You can refer to the chapter on Exercises to know how to practice these asanas.

Issues or Health Conditions	Beneficial Asanas
1. Abdomen and Buttocks (Toning)	Ardha Pawanmukthasana, Naukasana, Dhanurasana
2. Acidity	Pawanmuktasana, Kati Chakrasana, Brahma Mudra
3. Ailments of Back, Neck and Waist	Suptvajrasana, Bhujangasana, Triyak Bhujangasana
4. Arthritis	Tadasana, Gomukhasana, Bhadrasana
5. Appendicitis	Paschimottanasana, Vipreetkarni, Matsyasana
6. Body Stiffness	Paschimottanasana, Matsyendrasana, Dhanurasana
7. Bronchial Asthma	Matsyanasana, Vakrasana, Chakrasana
8. Bronchitis	Sarvangasana, Tadasana, Bhujangasana
9. Cervical Spondylosis	Brahma Mudra, Bhujangasana, Kati Chakrasana
10. Congestion	Matsyasana, Chakrasana,
11. Chronic Cough and Cold	Ushtrasana, Back bending Chakrasana, Vakrasana
12. Constipation	Pawanmuktasana, Ardh Halasana, Naukasana
13. Diabetes	Ardha Pawanmuktasana, Naukasana, Dhanurasana

(*Cont.*)

14.	Dyspepsia	Sarvangasana, Matsyasana, Shirshasana
15.	Eosinophilia	Bhujangasana, Sarpasana, Supine Naukasana
16.	Excess Fat Deposition	Ardhhalasana, Naukasana, Matsyanasana
17.	Flatulence and Gastric Problems	Pawanmuktasana, Naukasana, Shalabhasana
18.	Genital Diseases	Matysasana, Vipreetkarni, Suptvajrasana
19.	Headache	Pawanmuktasana, Brahma Mudra, Shirshasana
20.	Heart Disease	Ardha Pawanmuktasana, Ardha Halasana, Bhujangasana
21.	High Blood Pressure	Tadasana, Trikonasana, Kati Chakrasana
22.	Hip Joint Pain	Vakrasana, Matsyasana, Poorna Halasana
23.	Hypertension	Ardha Pawanmuktasana, Shavasana, Makrasana
24.	Hypertension	Naukasana, Shalabhasana, Dhanurasana
25.	Knee, Ankle and Joint Pain	Gomukhasana, Parvatasana, Paschimottanasana
26.	Low Blood Pressure	Pawanmuktasana, Kati Chakrasana, Matsyasana

(*Cont.*)

27.	Lumbar Pain	Kati Chakrasana, Shalabhasana, Supine Naukasana
28.	Mental Disorders	Shavasana, Vakrasana,
29.	Menstrual Disorders	Halasana, Sarvangasana, Matsyasana
30.	Migraine	Vipreetkarni, Sarvangasana, Shirshasana
31.	Piles	Ashwaschanchalasana, Vajrasana, Pawanmuktasana
32.	Problems related to Liver, Pancreas, Kidney and Bladder	Naukasana, Triyak Naukasana, Ushtrasana
33.	Problem related to Nervous System	Vrikshasana, Tadasana, Natrajasana
34.	Pyorrhoea	Simhasana, Matsyasana, Brahma Mudra
35.	Rheumatism	Paschimottanasana, Shalabhasana, Bhujangasana
36.	Sciatica Pain	Kati Chakrasana, Setubandhasana, Shalabhasana
37.	Spondylitis or Spinal Problems	Sarpasana, Bhujangasana, Supine Naukasana
38.	Tonsillitis	Ushtrasana, Simhasana, Matsyasana
39.	Urinary Tract Infection and related diseases	Bhadrasana, Vipreetkarni, Poorna Halasana

THINGS YOU SHOULD KNOW BEFORE DOING ASANAS

There are a few things that you should know about asanas. Please keep these in mind before you practice any of the above mentioned postures.

a. Children below 12 years of age should not practice asanas for long periods of time. Most of the postures are not suitable for young kids. Therefore these must be done under expert guidance only.
b. To gain maximum benefits, perform yoga every day for 30-45 minutes.
c. The best time to practice the postures would be in the morning, one hour after getting up from bed. Do not exercise immediately after waking up. Wait for some time before you start exercising.
d. Do not practice asanas if you are suffering from very high blood pressure, dizziness, or severe eye problems. Consult your doctor, if in doubt.
e. Perform the asanas early in the morning or early in the evening. Never exercise on a full stomach or directly after a meal. Wait for at least 3 hours after your meal, before starting the postures. After performing the asanas, there should be a gap of at least one hour before you have your meals. You can have a fruit or a glass of juice, one hour prior to and after the exercises.
f. Never take a hot shower bath immediately after yoga. You can bathe with lukewarm or cold water.
g. Asanas must be performed in a well-ventilated room. An open, clean, and peaceful space is preferable.

h. Spread a carpet or thick mat on the floor before performing asanas. You should not practice these on the bed or a hard floor.
i. Wear clean, loose, comfortable clothes. Undergarments should be worn while performing the postures.
j. Perform the asanas slowly without straining your body. Do not continue if you experience any sort of pain or discomfort.
k. Do not practice yoga during the first three days of menstruation and in the first three months of your pregnancy.
l. While performing standing postures make sure that your feet are firmly grounded and that your body weight is properly balanced.
m. While doing back bends, be very careful. Do not push yourself beyond limits and hurt your spine.
n. Inhale while bending backwards and exhale while bending forward.
o. Increase your repetitions slowly and steadily. Be patient and try not to rush into doing every posture at once. Building stamina is an important component of asanas. Do not try to overdo any particular posture. If you are unable to do a specific asana, practice regularly till you achieve your target posture.
p. Practice regularly for best results. You can perform the asanas six days a week. Make sure that you breathe properly through your nose.
q. Focus on your body and breath. Don't stretch yourself beyond your capacity.

Now that we have discussed the benefits of asanas and how you can incorporate it in your daily life, let us go to the next chapter which deals with one of my favourite asanas. This particular exercise works wonders for your body. And what's more, all my clients love it! Do you want to know which one it is? Turn the page and find it out yourself.

Yoga Quiz Answers:

1 c	6 c
2 b	7 a
3 d	8 c
4 a	9 d
5 b	10 a

SURYANAMASKAR: SUN IT UP

I am sure a lot of you want to have a body like Kareena's—perfectly toned muscles and curves to die for. So what's the secret behind Bebo's sylph like figure? Any guesses? Of course, it is Suryanamaskar. Most of you must have heard about it. So what actually is Suryanamaskar? How does it work for our overall fitness? Let's find out.

Suryanamaskar makes the entire body flexible and prepares it for asanas. Popularly known as sun salutations, it is an elegant sequence of twelve postures completed as one continuous cycle. If you do it in a flow in the proper way it is one of the most rhythmic and beautiful exercises. All postures respond to each other and help stretch the body in different ways through rhythmic breathing. Suryanamaskar reduces stiffness, rejuvenates the body, and invigorates the mind. Everyday practice also helps in trimming the waist and makes the joints and spine supple.

THE BASICS

Suryanamaskar is an age-old practice that involves reverence to the Sun deity. It is ideally done in the morning at the break of dawn, facing the East by offering homage to the Sun through different postures and salutations.

The twelve stages that constitute one Suryanamaskar cycle are:

a. Namaskar Mudra
b. Back bending Chakrasana
c. Padahastasana
d. Ashwa Sanchalanasana
e. Santolanasana
f. Shashtanga Mudra
g. Sarpasana
h. Parvatasana
i. Ashwa Sanchalanasana
j. Padahastasana
k. Back bending Chakrasana
l. Namaskar Mudra

Suryanamaskar can do miracles to your body—transform you into a new you. Try it out for just 15 days and you will notice the difference. In fact it is what I call 'a complete package'—a spiritually elevating exercise involving the body, mind, and breathing which improves our knowledge of our inner self. If you really want to look and feel good, just kick start your day with Suryanamaskar. Two consecutive sets of twelve poses and you complete one round. So let's get started.

DO IT RIGHT

1. Posture 1—Namaskar Mudra:

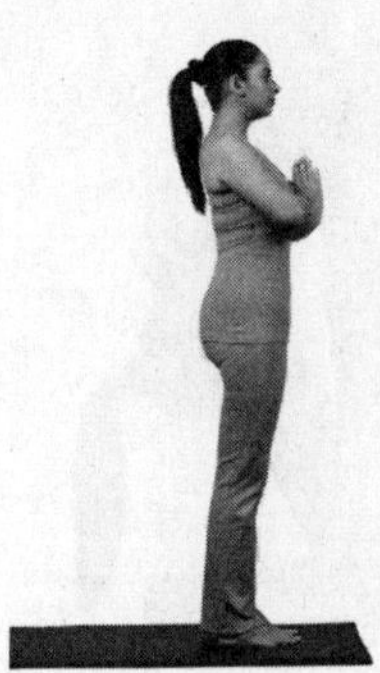

Stand straight with your feet together and hands by the side. Now bring your palms together close to your chest in Namaskar Mudra, breathing normally.

2. Posture 2—Back bending Chakrasana:

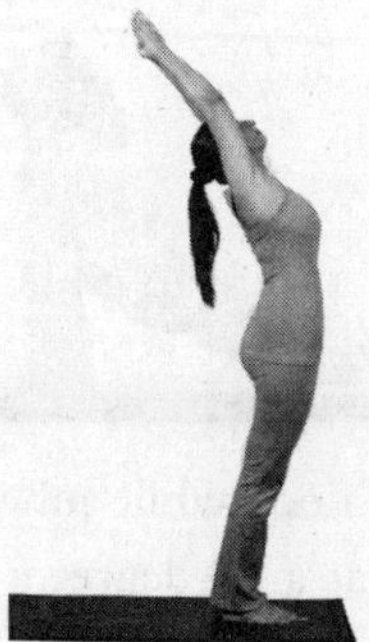

Inhale and raise your hands upwards. Now arch your back and stretch your arms upwards as far back as you can. Once you are in this position, breathe normally.

3. Posture 3—Padahastasana:

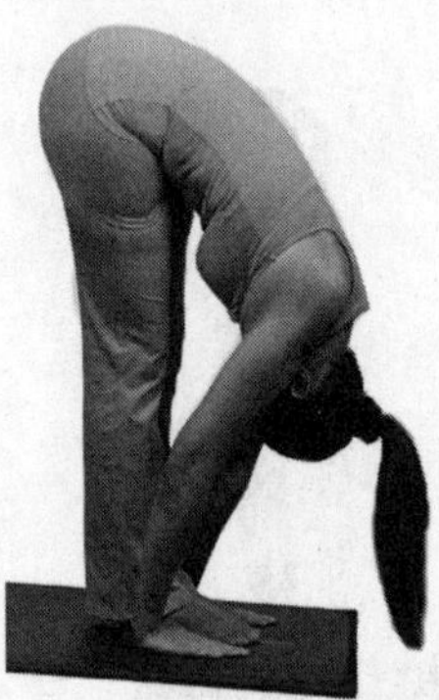

Exhale and bend forward, touching your toes with your hands without bending the knees. Look downwards and breathe normally once you are in this posture.

4. Posture 4—Ashwa Sanchalanasana:

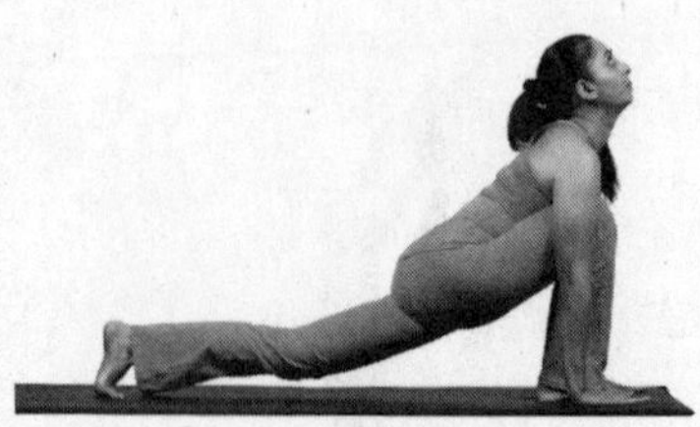

Place your palms on the floor while inhaling, bend the right leg between your hands at a 90-degree angle from the floor, then stretch the left leg backwards. Now arch your back and look upwards, breathing normally.

5. Posture 5—Santolanasana:

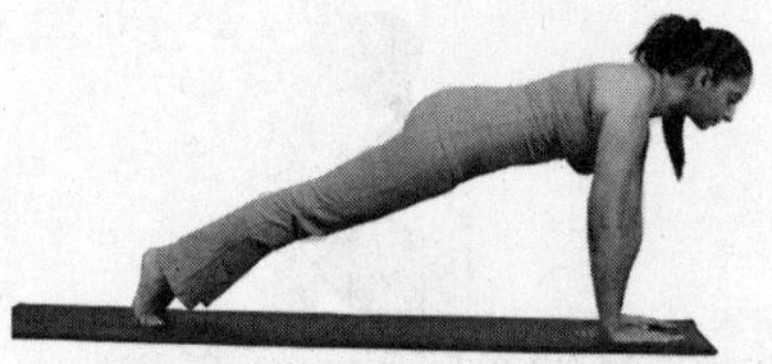

Exhale and place your right leg behind, so that it is in line with your left leg. Make sure your hands are aligned below with your shoulders. The shoulders, back, and hips should be in one straight line. Breathe normally when you are in this posture.

6. Posture 6—Shashtanga Mudra:

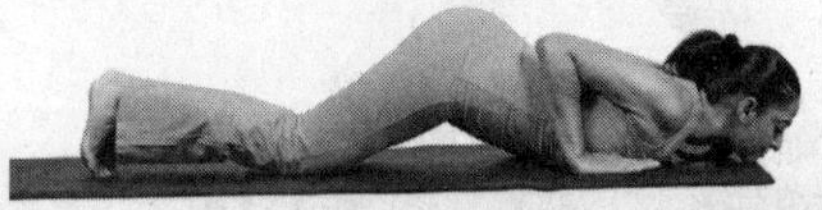

Bend the elbows, chin, chest and knees towards the floor. Tuck the elbows on the sides and close to the body. Now raise the hips upwards, breathing normally.

7. Posture 7—Sarpasana:

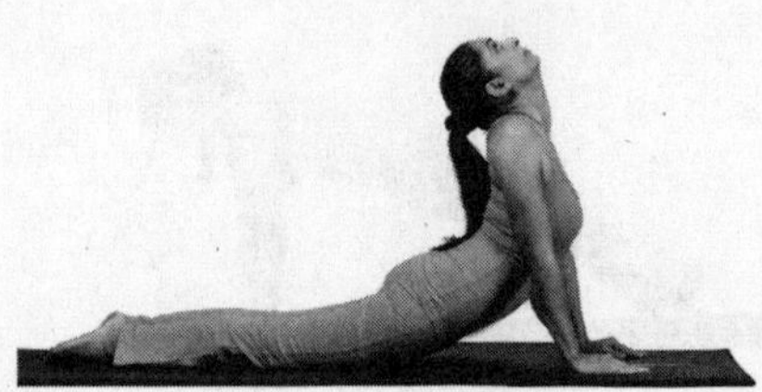

Inhale and raise the upper body with the shoulders bending backwards and the chin upwards. The waist should touch the floor. Once in the final posture, breathe normally.

8. Posture 8—Parvatasana:

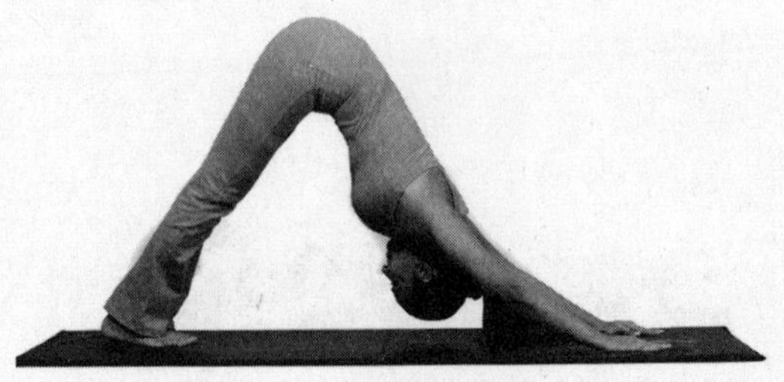

Exhale and raise the hips upwards, pushing the upper body behind and touching the heels to the floor. Keep your knees straight and neck facing downwards looking at the navel region, once in posture, breathe normally.

9. Posture 9—Ashwa Sanchalanasana:

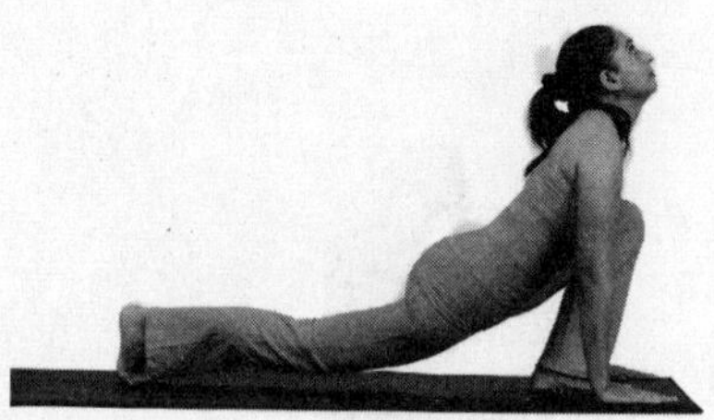

Inhale while placing your left leg forward and in between the hands. Now arch your back, press the chin upwards, keeping the palms flat on the floor. Breathe normally once you are in this posture.

10. Posture 10—Padahastasana:

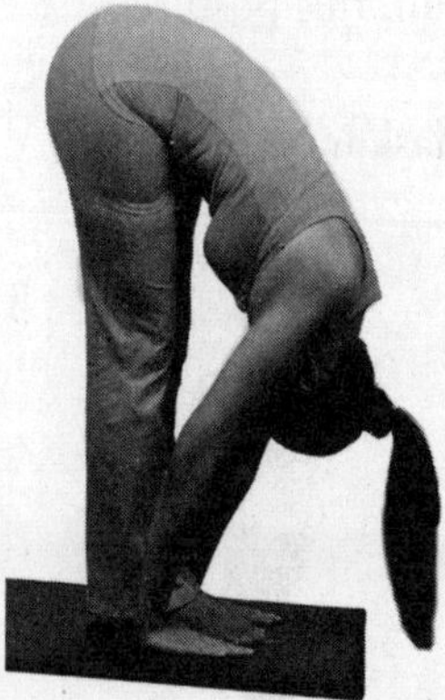

Bring your left leg forward towards your right leg, keeping the knees straight. Now with the palms touching the toe and the neck relaxed. Once you attain this posture, breathe normally.

11. Posture 11—Back bending Chakrasana:

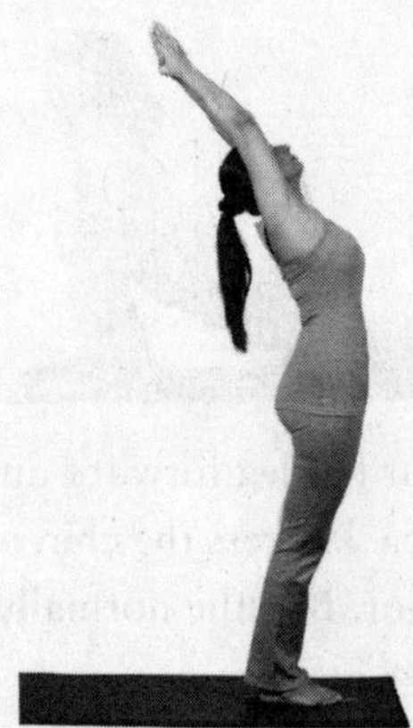

Bring your palms together, inhale and raise the hands and the upper body upwards while arching your back. Breathe normally once you attain this posture.

12. Posture 12—Namaskar Mudra:

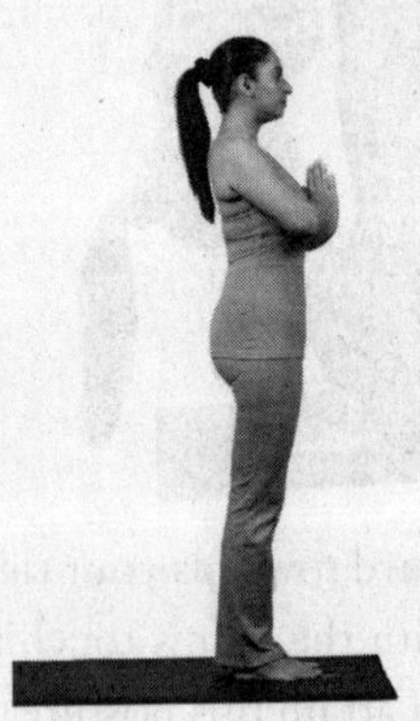

Come back to the starting position slowly while exhaling.

Why do I swear by Suryanamaskar?

Suryanamaskar, like I said, is a holistic exercise that provides physical, mental, and spiritual health benefits. It is a complete body workout that helps in detoxification, weight loss, making skin radiant, and keeping stress at bay. Months of gymning, dieting, and working out will not really help as much as this simple exercise. Here are some of its benefits:

a. It is an easy and pleasant way of starting the day. You will feel fresh and rejuvenated after practising the postures.
b. It does not cause any kind of sprain or injury. So it is advisable for people of all age groups.
c. It relieves tension and stress, and has a soothing effect on the mind.
d. It works wonders on the muscles making them strong and supple.
e. It helps fight insomnia and sleep disorders. Combating mental disorders and depression also becomes easy.
f. Joints, ligaments, and the skeletal system are strengthened by it. It also helps in maintaining balance, good posture, and poise.
g. It increases concentration power by stimulating the faculties of mind. You can in fact work better as it boosts your ability to focus.
h. It helps control hunger.
i. Makes the skin look radiant and younger.
j. It is good for the heart and stimulates the cardiovascular system by oxygenating blood.
k. It is the only exercise that provides workout for the entire body.

l. Digestive and nervous systems function in resonance.
m. It tones the body and cuts down body fat. It can easily reduce abdominal fat.
n. It supports the respiratory and lymphatic system.
o. Endocrine system that includes thyroid, parathyroid, adrenal, and pituitary glands as well as testes and ovaries, also function properly.

Tips for doing Suryanamaskar

Even though Suryanamaskar is appropriate for every age group, a few things should be kept in mind:

- The best time to perform suryanamaskar is in the morning on an empty stomach. However you can do it at any time of the day after 4 hours of having a meal.
- Clean and quiet environment is ideal for this exercise. It should preferably be done facing the sun.
- Do not wear tight fitting clothes or uncomfortable shoes. Wear light cotton clothes and sports shoes.
- If you are used to having tea or coffee as soon as you wake up in the morning, perform the asanas after half an hour.
- Healthy, balanced diet should be followed throughout the day. Do not overeat.
- Avoid Suryanamaskar during the first three days of your menstruation.
- If pregnant, you should not do Suryanamaskars.
- Try the postures only after consulting your doctor, if you are suffering from high blood pressure or any heart disease.
- Try not to perform the asanas if you have severe headache or backache.
- Consult an expert if you feel any kind of discomfort or pain.

POSTURES SIMPLIFIED

Each posture of Suryanamaskar has a distinctive function. From body balancing to blood circulation, these asanas are extremely helpful. Let us understand the benefits of each one so as to have a complete picture.

POSTURE 1—NAMASKAR MUDRA

a. Maintains the balance of the body.
b. Stimulates the respiratory system.
c. Exercises the shoulders, back, and neck muscles.
d. Helps develop good posture.

POSTURE 2—BACK BENDING CHAKRASANA

a. Promotes digestion.
b. Strengthens chest muscles.
c. Expands the lungs and opens the heart chakra.
d. Exercises arms and shoulder muscles.
e. Tones the spine.
f. Increases back and hip flexibility.
g. Promotes balance.

POSTURE 3—PADAHASTASANA

a. Promotes good blood circulation.
b. Tones abdominal tract.
c. Makes the waist and spine flexible.
d. Stretches leg and back muscles.
e. Stimulates spinal nerves.
f. Lymphatic system is also stimulated.
g. It is beneficial for the functioning of the liver.

POSTURE 4—ASHWA SANCHALANASANA

a. Strengthens hand, legs, and wrist muscles.
b. Exercises the spinal cord.
c. Massages abdominal organs.
d. Helps develop confidence.
e. Makes the neck muscles flexible.

POSTURE 5—SANTOLANASANA

a. Strengthens the arms and wrists.
b. Maintains body posture.
c. Stimulates blood's circulation to the brain.
d. Strengthens the heart.
e. Relieves tension.

POSTURE 6—SHASHTANGA MUDRA

a. Strengthens the core muscles.
b. Expands the chest muscles.
c. Waist and spine become flexible.
d. Releases tension from the neck and spine.
e. Helps reduce abdominal fat.

POSTURE 7—SARPASANA

a. Makes the spine flexible.
b. Increases blood's circulation to the abdominal area.
c. Relieves constipation.
d. Stimulates spinal nerves.
e. Tones muscles.
f. Reduces fat.

POSTURE 8—PARVATASANA

a. Good for spine and waist muscles.
b. Strengthens the arms.
c. Improves blood circulation.
d. Relieves stress.

POSTURE 9—ASHWA SANCHALANASANA

a. Strengthens the legs.
b. Abdomen is massaged by it.
c. Improves flexibility of the body.

POSTURE 10—PADAHASTASANA

a. Promotes blood circulation.
b. Abdominal tract remains healthy and well regulated.
c. Strengthens the back.
d. Stimulates the spinal nerves.

POSTURE 11—BACK BENDING CHAKRASANA

a. Promotes body's balance.
b. Expands the abdominal viscera.
c. Tones the spine.
d. Expands the lungs.
e. Helps in proper digestion.

POSTURE 12—NAMASKAR MUDRA

a. Body is balanced.
b. Helps maintain poise.
c. Exercises the shoulder and neck muscles.

With this we come to the end of the chapter on my favourite yoga exercise, Suryanamaskar. Let me share something with you. It's not only me! A lot of my friends and clients swear by it and do it while travelling, in hotel rooms, or even on the beach. It's a complete, holistic, and natural way to body care that is easy to get addicted to. And this is a kind of addiction that we should have. Why don't you try it out and write to me about it?

EXERCISES

Some of you might wonder why I have written one whole chapter on the description of asanas, outlined the procedures in detail and tried to explain ways of doing it correctly. The answer is simple. I want the book to be as practical and useful as possible. I want you to be able to actually do the asanas and hence I have also included pictures as there is nothing better than visuals to show how to do exercises. This was also a feedback I got from many of my readers. I hope you will find value in this and use it to make a difference in your well-being.

1. Ardha Halasana (Half Plough Pose):

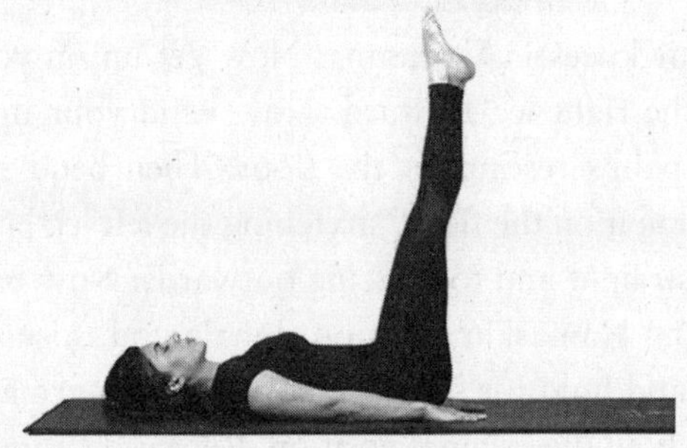

Lie in supine position with your feet together, hands at the side of your body and palms facing downwards. Inhale and contract your lower abdomen muscles. While exhaling, raise both your legs up to 90 degrees from the floor. Keep moving your legs from 90 degrees to 0 degrees while inhaling down and exhaling up, with lower abdominal contractions.

2. Ardha Kapotasana (Half Pigeon Pose):

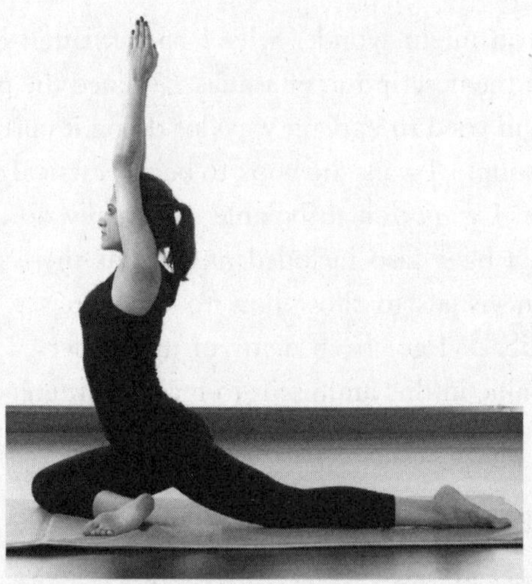

Sit on your knees in Vajrasana. Now get up on your knees, and put the right leg forward. Now bend your upper body with the palms resting on the floor. Then bend your right knee putting it on the floor, stretching the left leg behind with the knee straight and toes facing outwards. Now balance the body in the Namaskar position. Inhale and raise the hands upwards and hold for some time, breathing normally. Come back slowly to the original position. Repeat the same with the other side.

3. Ardha Matsyendrasana (Half Spinal Twist Pose):

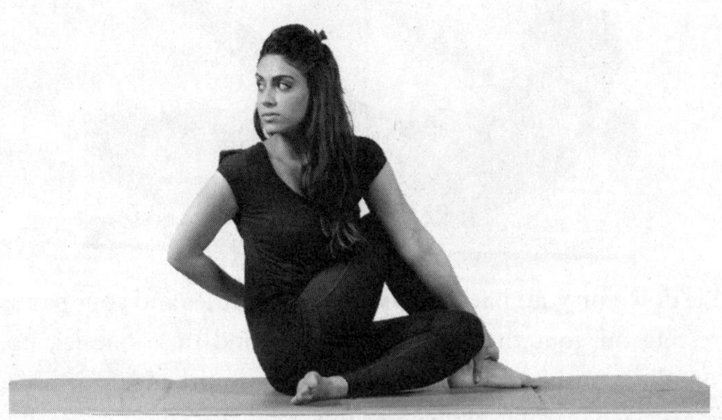

Sit on the floor with both the legs extended together, hands by the side of the body, and palms resting on the floor. Now bend the right leg at the knee, and slowly put the right heel at the perineum. Then, bending the left leg, bring it from above the right knee and place it by the side, on the floor. The knee of the left leg should face the ceiling. Now bring the right hand on the left side, over the left knee and hold your left ankle with your right hand. Twisting the body to the left side, look backwards, and place the left hand on the floor close to your spine with the elbow straightened. Hold for some time, breathing normally, and come back slowly to the original position. Repeat the same with the other side and the other leg.

4. Ardha Naukasana (Half Boat Pose):

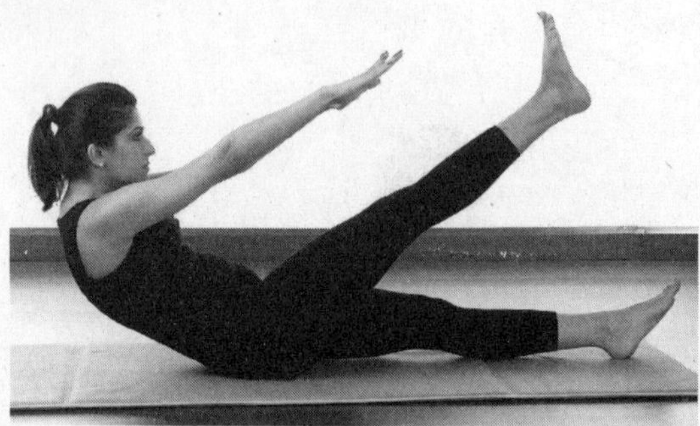

Lie down on your back with your feet together and your palms resting on your thighs. Inhale slowly and raise one leg up, simultaneously raising the upper body and hands upwards, towards the toe. Hold for some time while breathing normally. Then come down slowly to the original position and repeat with the other leg.

5. Ardha Pawanmuktasana (Half Wind Relieving Pose):

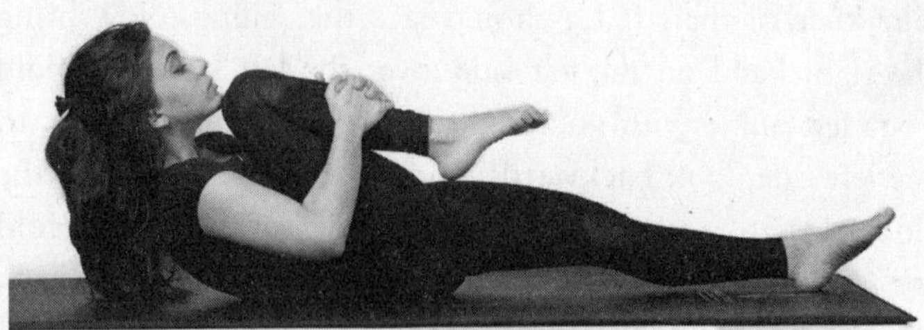

Lie in a supine position with legs together, hands by the side, and palms resting on the floor. Bend right leg slowly towards your chest, hold your right knee and press it well towards the chest. Then while exhaling, raise the chin up and try to touch the right knee, hold this for some time while breathing normally. Then come back to the original position and repeat the same with the other leg.

6. Ardha Shalabhasana (Half Locust Pose):

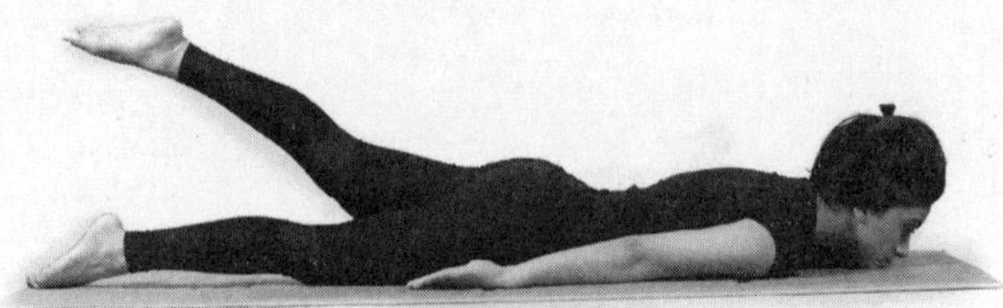

Lie in a prone position and bring your legs together, toes pointing outward, hands by the side of the body, and forehead touching the floor. Then slowly raise the right leg without bending at the knee. Do not tilt the pelvis. Hold for some time with normal breathing, come back to the original position, and repeat the same with the other leg.

7. Ardha Triyak Naukasana (Half-bent Boat Pose):

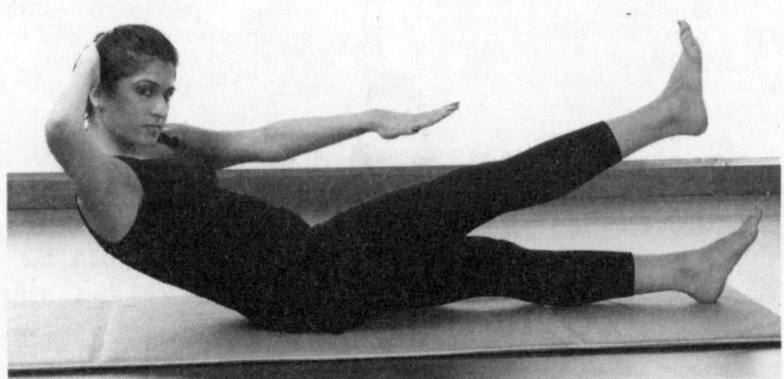

Lie on your back with feet together and palms resting on your thighs. Inhale first and while exhaling slowly raise your right leg up as well as your upper body while twisting your upper body to the right side. Now place your right hand behind your head. Hold for some time, breathing normally. Come down slowly to the original position and do the same with the other leg.

8. Ashwin Mudra:

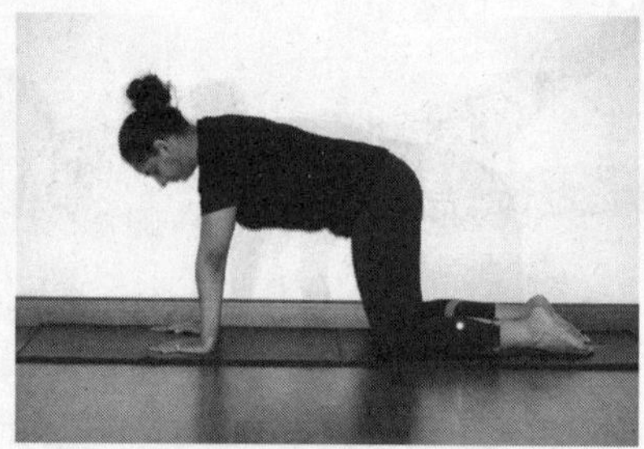

In cat pose, while inhaling, expand your anus muscles outwards and while exhaling, contract your anus muscles inwards. Repeat this 10 to 15 times. Relax your body and breathe normally.

9. Bhadrasana (Gracious Pose):

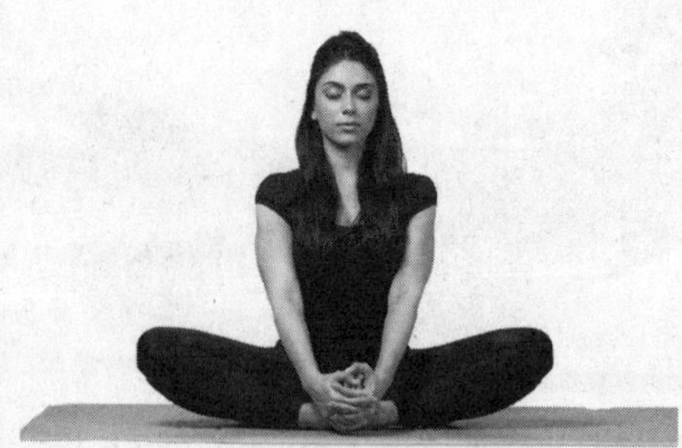

Sit on the floor with your legs extended in front of you, hands by the side, and back straight. Now slowly bend your knees downwards while placing the soles of your feet together. Hold your toes with the hands, and slowly move your knees up and down a few time to loosen the muscles of your inner thighs. Then hold your feet with both hands and push your knees towards the floor. Hold for some time breathing normally and then slowly come back to the original position.

10. Bhujangasana (Lying Cobra Pose):

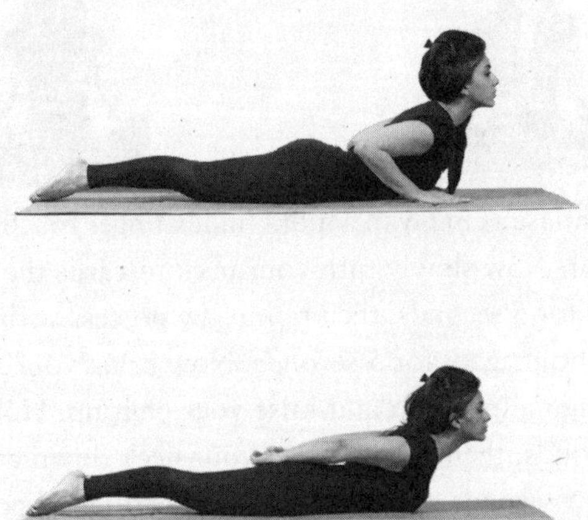

Lie in a prone position, legs together, toes together and pointing outwards, hands by the side of the body, palms facing upwards, and forehead on the floor. Now bend hands from the elbows, place the palms on the floor near each side of the shoulder. The thumb should be under the armpit. Inhale and raise your chin, turn your head upwards as much as possible, and raise your upper body up to the navel. Try to keep the palms off the floor by tucking the elbows close to the body. Hold this for some time breathing normally, then while exhaling come down to the original position.

11. Brahma Mudra:

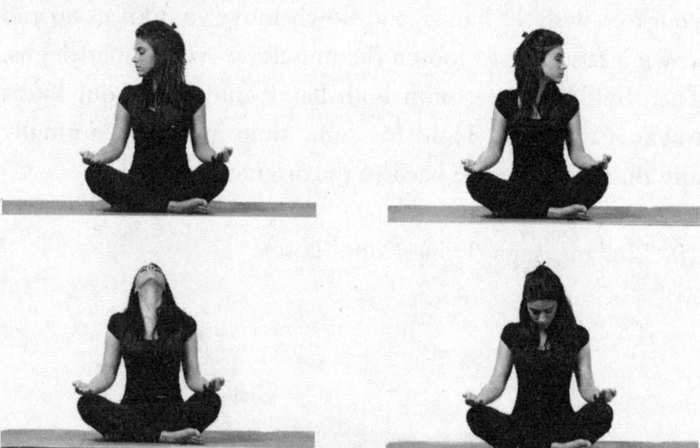

Sit in Padmasana in Gyan Mudra (index finger touching the tip of thumb). Now slowly turn your neck towards the right side and hold for 5 seconds, then repeat the process with the other side and hold again for 5 seconds. Now bring your neck back to the original position and raise your chin up. Hold it there for 5 seconds, then slowly bring your neck down and hold it there for 5 seconds and come back to the original position.

12. Chakrasana (Wheel Pose):

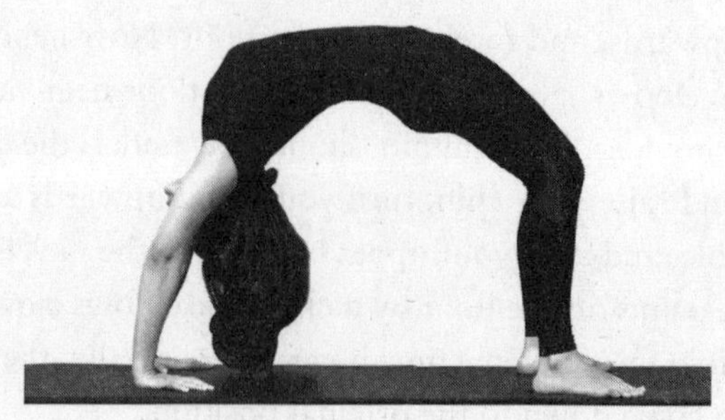

Lie in a supine position, legs together, hands by the side, palms facing the floor. Now bend your legs at the knees, and place your feet apart on the floor close to the butt. Place your hands under the shoulder, palms facing down, and elbows upwards. Slowly lift the waist and upper body upwards with the help of the hands, while keeping the neck muscles relaxed. Hold this for some time breathing normally. While coming back first bend the elbows, put the head on the floor, then shoulder, upper back, mid-back, lower back, and finally place the butt on the floor and come back to the original position.

13. Chakrasana (Side Bending):

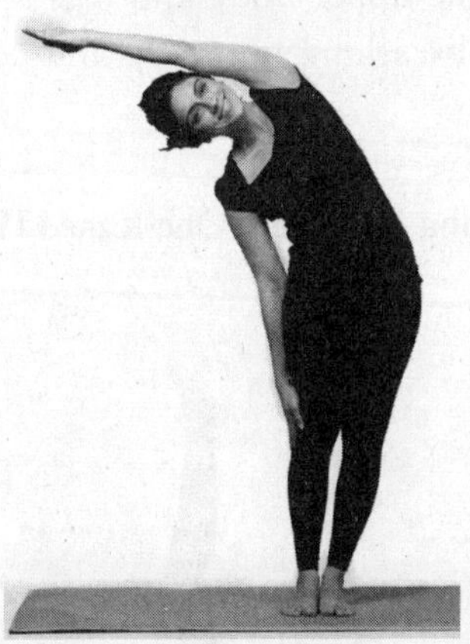

While standing, put your feet together with the hands on the side. Now raise your right hand up and stretch while bending your body towards the left side. Hold for some time, and come back to the original position. Repeat it with the other side.

14. Dhanurasana (The Bow Pose):

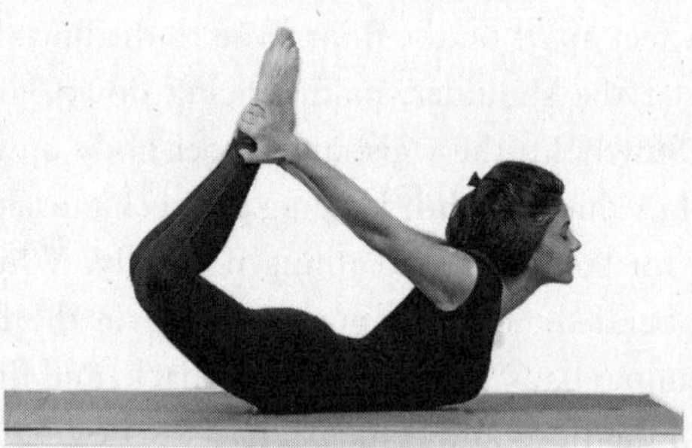

Lie in a prone position facing the floor, feet together, hands by the side and forehead on the floor. Now bend your knees, hold the ankles with both hands and, while inhaling, raise the upper body and legs up together. Hold for some time, breathing normally and come back to the original position.

15. Ek Pada Ardha Halasana (One-legged Half Plough Pose):

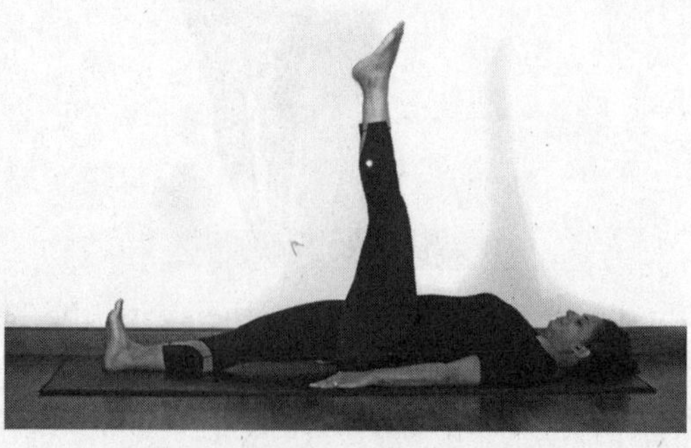

Lie in a supine position with your legs together and hands by the side. While exhaling, raise the right leg upto 60 degrees from the floor then inhale and come back. Repeat the same with the left leg. Keep repeating this with alternate legs for some time.

16. Ek Pada Hasta Santolanasana (Hand and Leg Upwards):

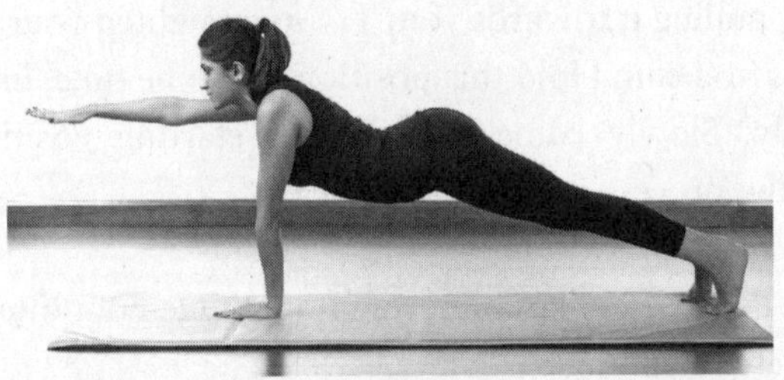

Sit in cat pose, straighten your knees, move the shoulders forward and the buttock downwards until the body is straight like in position no. 5 of Suryanamaskar. Now raise the hand parallel to the ear. Hold for some time, breathing normally. Then slowly repeat the same with the other side.

17. Ek Pada Ugrasana (One Foot Fierce Pose):

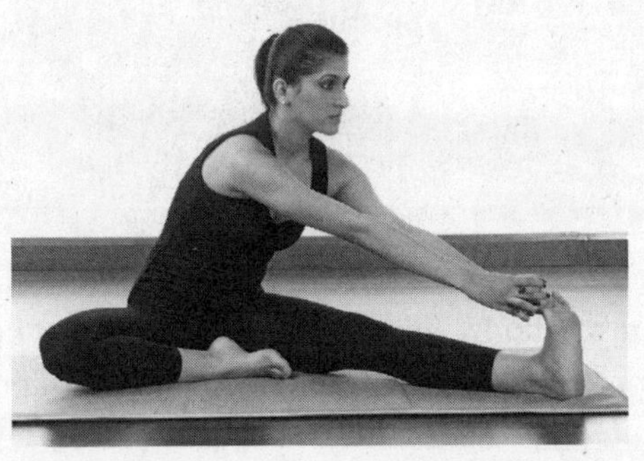

Sit straight on the floor, stretching both legs together in front of you with palms resting on the floor. Now slowly widen the legs as much as you can bending slightly forward. Bend your right leg at the knee with the help of your right hand, pushing your right foot under your left thigh. Now slowly raise your hands upwards, bend forward and try to hold your big toe, pulling it towards you. Try to straighten your back as much as you can. Hold this position for some time, breathing normally. Slowly come back to the starting position and repeat the process with the other leg.

18. Ek Pada Uttan Paschimottanasana (One Foot Intense Leg Stretch Bending):

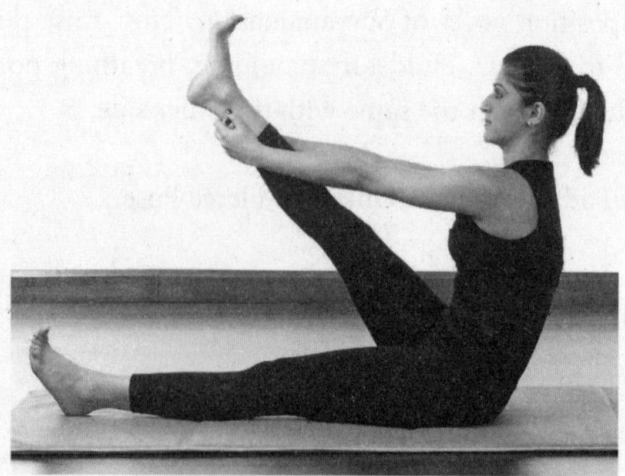

Sit on the floor with the legs straight in the front, hands by the side of the body, and palms resting on the floor. Now bend the right knee and hold the right ankle with both hands, keeping the right knee straight while raising it up as much as you can. Keep your back straight and hold it there, breathing normally. Now slowly come back to the normal position and repeat the process with the other leg.

19. Ek Pada Vyaghrasana (One Foot King Pigeon Posture):

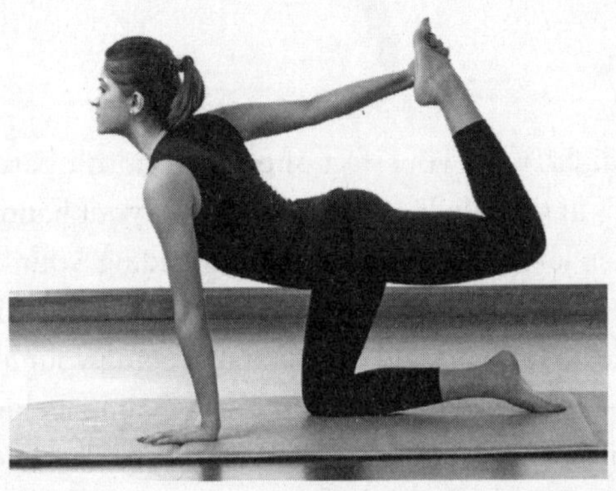

Sit on the floor with palms resting on the floor and your knees touching the ground like in cat pose. Place your hands under your shoulders. Your knees should be apart at the same level. Now raise your right leg upwards without applying pressure on your back. Bend your right leg at the knee, taking your right hand behind trying to hold your right foot. Now while holding your right foot, raise your head backwards and raise your right leg further, as much as you can. Hold this position, breathing normally. Slowly come back to the starting position. Repeat the posture with the other leg.

20. Front Kick:

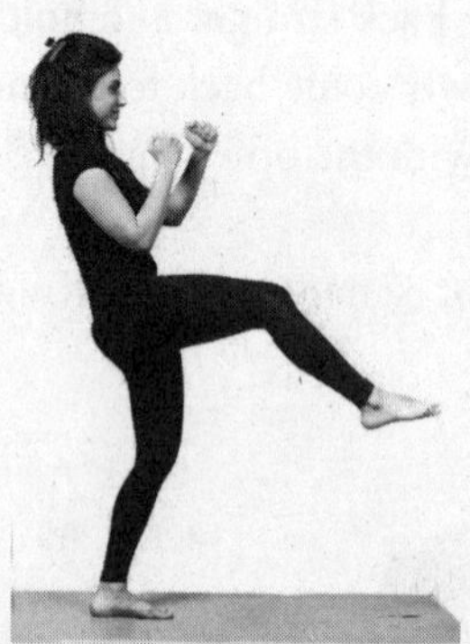

Stand straight with your feet shoulder width apart, keeping your hands at the side of your body. Stretch your hands forward at shoulder level and close your fist bending your elbows at 90 degrees upwards. Now take your right leg behind, bend your left leg a little bit and inhale first keeping your abdominal muscles tight and kick forward while exhaling as high as you can. Keep moving with this motion, going back while inhaling and kicking forward while exhaling. Repeat with the other leg.

21. Garudasana (Eagle Pose):

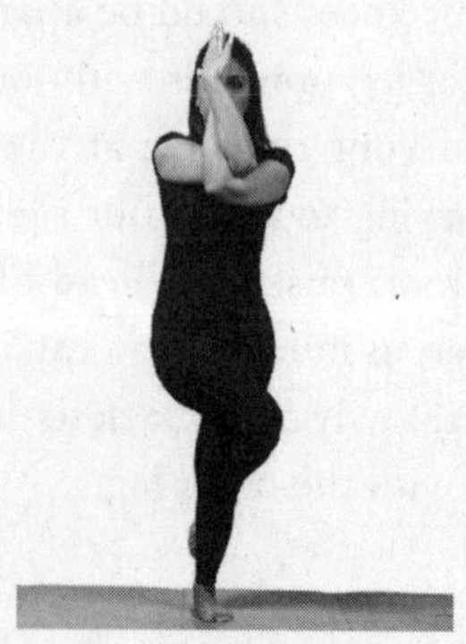

This asana is done in the standing position with your feet together, and hands by the side. Bend your knees slightly, and entangle your right leg over the left leg. Similarly, entangle your right hand with your left hand and bring it to chest level, balancing the body on one leg. Hold for some time, breathing normally. Follow the same with the other leg and hand.

22. Gomukhasana(Cow Face Pose):

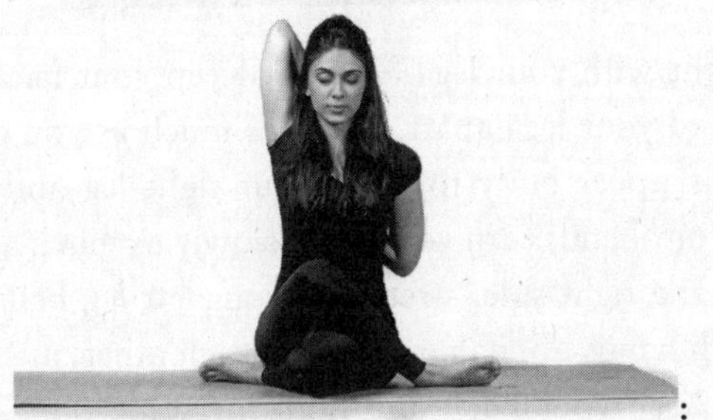
:

Sit on the floor stretching your legs forward. Bend both your knees slightly. Place your left leg under your right thigh and take your right leg over your left leg, making sure both your knees are under each other. Now take your right hand with elbow facing the ceiling behind your back with your fingers facing downwards. Now take your left hand behind your back. Try holding both your palms together, making sure your entire back is straight and aligned with your neck. Breathe normally once you are in this posture. Repeat the same with the other leg and hand. Hold for some time and come back to the original position.

23. Hanumanasana (Monkey Pose):

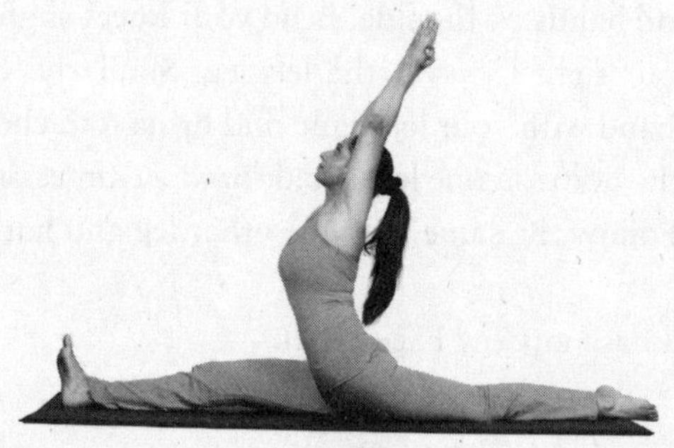

Sit straight with your legs forward. Keep your back straight and spread your legs apart slowly as much as you can. Now turn your upper body towards your right leg and with the help of your hands turn your body slowly as much as you can towards the right side, stretching your left leg behind. Now raise both hands up, palms touching each other, in Namaskar Mudra. Arch your back and hold for some time breathing normally. Do the same with the other leg.

24. Jalandhara Bandha (can be done while inhaling and exhaling):

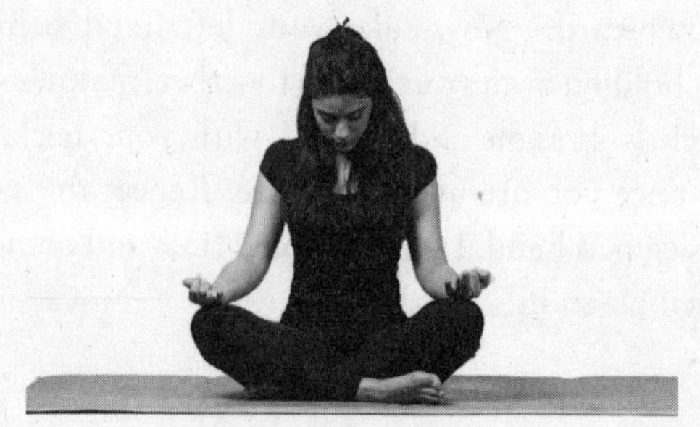

Sit in any meditative or comfortable position on the floor with your back straight and shoulders relaxed. Inhale slowly, hold your breath, and gradually drop your chin down as much as you can. Hold for as long as you can. Now slowly get your chin back to the original position and exhale through your nose. Sit in any meditative or comfortable position on the floor with your back straight and shoulders relaxed. Inhale slowly through your nose and exhale holding your breath out. Drop your chin down as much as you can and hold for as long as you can. Lift your chin back gradually to the original position and inhale slowly through your nose.

25. Jumping Jack:

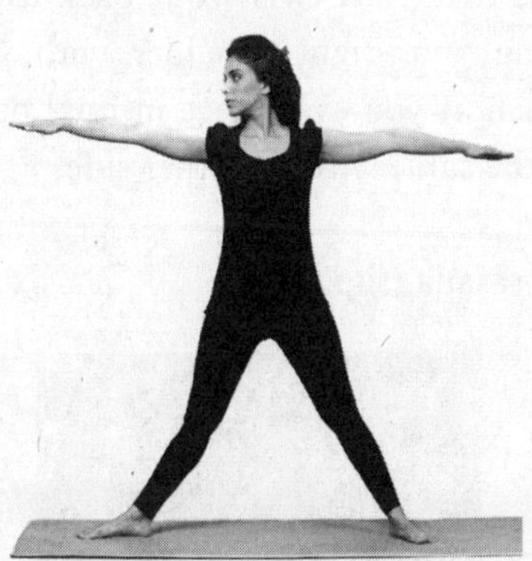

Stand straight with your hands by your side. Inhale and raise your hands up while jumping and keep your feet apart. Now exhale while bringing your hands down and bring your feet together at the same time. Repeat 15 to 20 times.

26. Kati Chakrasana (standing):

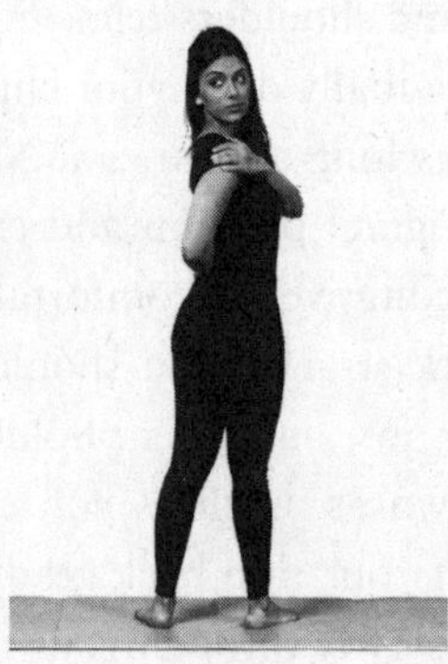

Stand straight with your feet shoulder width apart, keeping your hands at the side of your body. Now take your right hand behind on your lower back and keep your left hand on your right shoulder. Now twist your back towards the right side by pushing your right shoulder with your left hand, twisting as much as you can. Once in final position, breathe normally. Do the same with the other side.

27. Kati Chakrasana (supine):

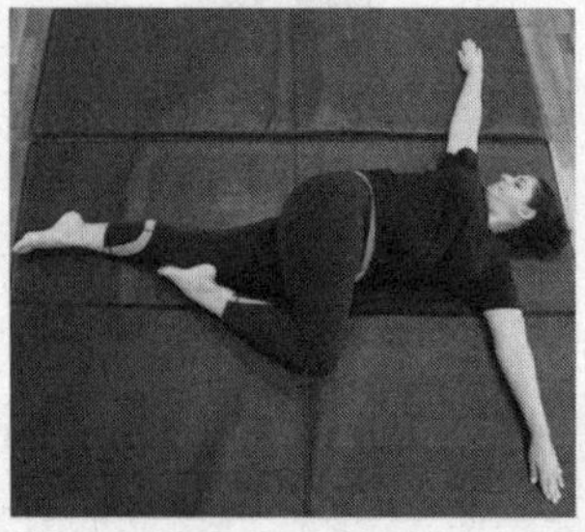

Lie in supine position, with both legs together and palms facing on the floor. Then spread your arms shoulder level apart. Bending your right knee, put your right foot on the left thigh. Right knee facing upwards, slowly bring your right knee towards the left side while twisting your back towards the right side and neck to the opposite side. Hold for some time breathing normally and come back to the original position. Repeat the same on the other side.

28. Lunges:

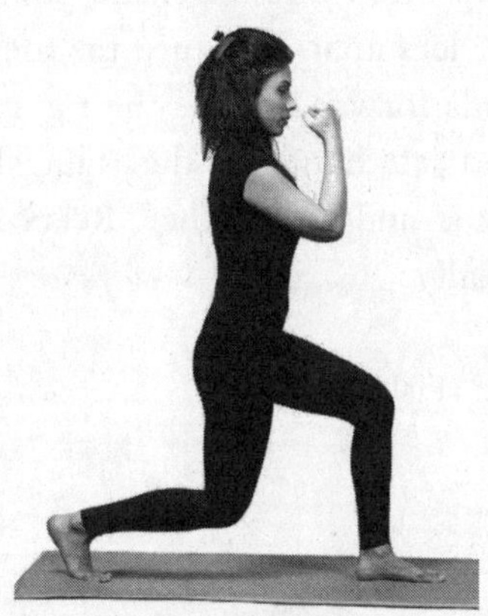

Stand straight with your feet shoulder width apart, keeping your hands at the side of your body. Stretch your hands forward at shoulder level and close your fist bending your elbows at 90 degrees upwards. Take your right leg behind, 2 feet away from your left leg. Bend both knees together making sure your right knee is off the floor and the left knee is not beyond your toes. In this position keep your back straight and keep moving while inhaling down and exhaling up. (Precaution: people with any knee problem shouldn't attempt this.) Do the same with the other leg.

29. Makarasana (Relaxing Pose):

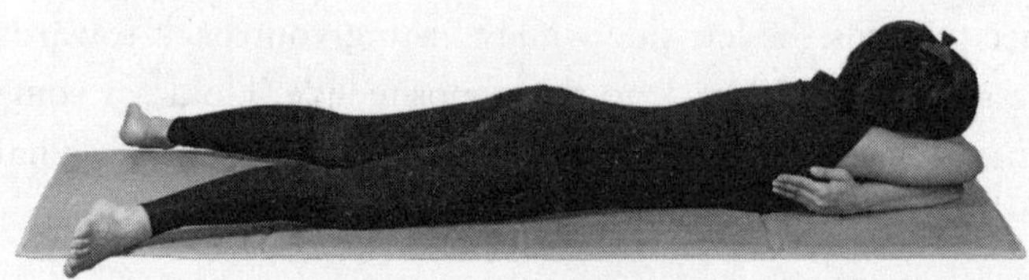

Lie in prone position, feet together, hands by the side, palms facing upwards and forehead touching the floor. Now spread the legs apart and turn the toes sideways, then stretch the hands forward. Place the right hand under the left armpit, and left hand on the right shoulder making sure one elbow is under the other. Relax in this position, breathing normally.

30. Matsyasana (Fish Pose):

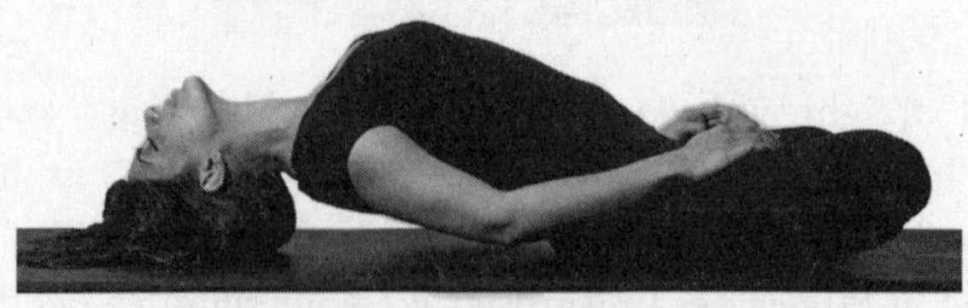

Sit in Padmasana. Taking your elbow's support, lie on your back slowly. Now bend your head backwards and touch it to the ground, while stretching your mid-back. Hold your toes with your index finger and keep the elbows on the ground at the same time. Hold for some time, breathing normally and come back to the original position.

31. Moola Bandha (Root Lock):

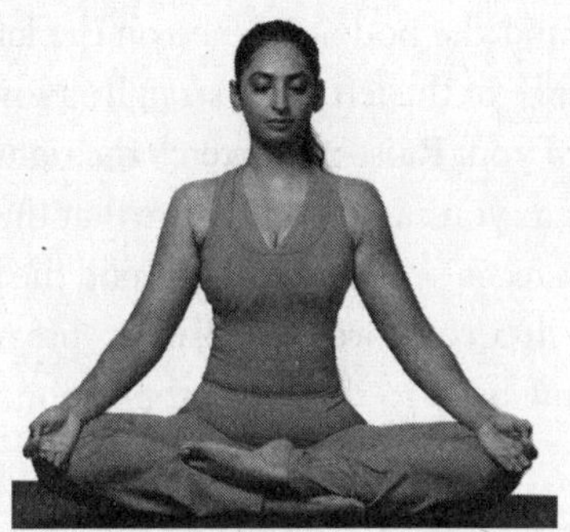

Sit in Padmasana or any meditative pose with your back straight, shoulders relaxed and sit in gyan mudra. Inhale deeply and slowly exhale and while exhaling contract your pelvic region as long as you can. Now slowly inhale and release the pelvic contraction. Breathing normally. Remain in this position for some time. Repeat 3-4 times.

32. Natrajasana (King of Dance Pose):

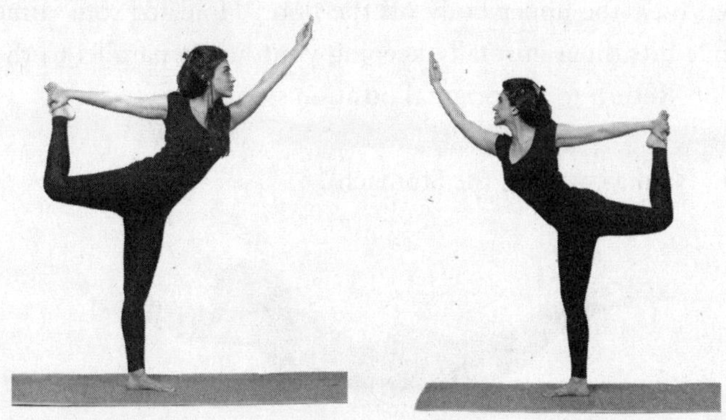

Stand straight with your feet together, and hands by the side of your thighs. Bend the right knee, holding the ankle with the right hand behind the body. Balance on the left leg and make sure that the knee of the left leg is straight. Now raise your left hand in front of you. Raise and stretch the right leg backwards slowly, as high as you can, making sure that the right hip is not twisted and the leg is raised directly behind the body. Hold this for some time in a comfortable position, breathing normally, and slowly come back to the original position.

33. Naukasana (Boat Pose on the Back):

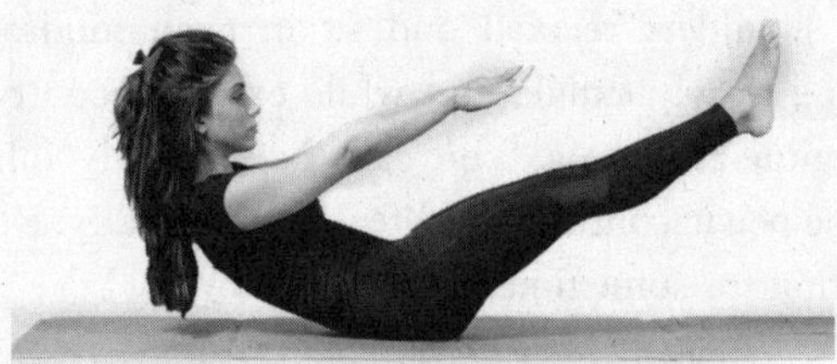

Lie down on your back with your feet together and your palms resting on your thighs. Inhale and raise both legs up, then raise the upper body off the floor. Hold for some time while breathing normally keeping your hands parallel to the floor. Return to the original position slowly.

34. Naukasana (On the Stomach):

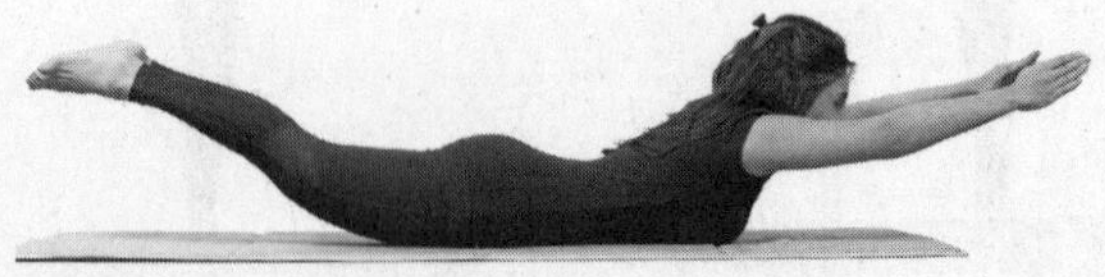

Lie down on your stomach with feet together, hands by the sides of the body, palms resting on the floor. Slowly bring both your hands parallel to your ears, making sure that the feet are together and the toes facing outwards. Now, slowly inhale and raise your upper and lower body together at the same time, making sure the arms keep touching the ears at all times. Once your body is in this boat like posture, hold it there and breathe normally. Slowly come back to the starting position.

35. Niralambasana (The Pillar Pose):

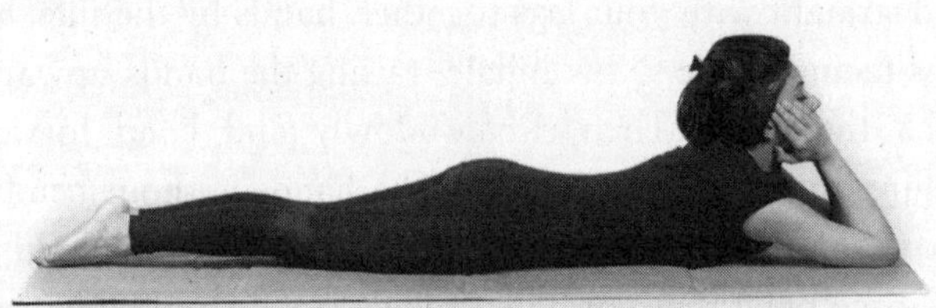

Lie in a prone position with your forehead on the floor, hands by the side, legs together, and toes pointed outwards. Slowly stretch the arms forward, and bend the elbows raising the head upwards. Place the chin on the palms, with your fingers touching the cheeks, making sure the elbows are together. Hold this for some time breathing normally. Then slowly come back to the original position.

36. Pada Hastasana (Feet and Hands Posture):

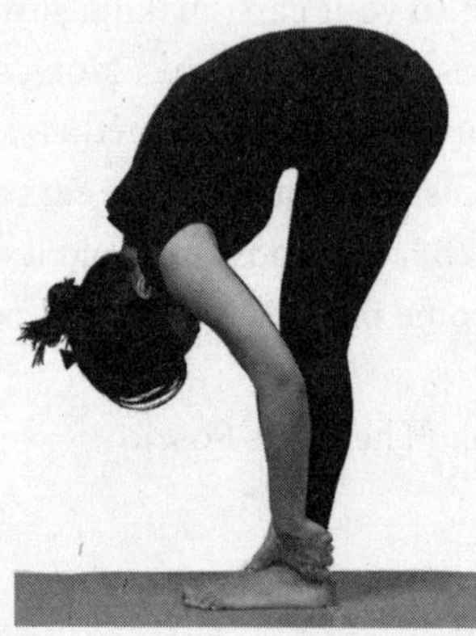

Stand straight with your legs together, hands by the side, and palms facing inside. Now inhale, raising the hands upwards, stretch the body. Then exhale slowly and bend forward touching the floor, or toes, with the hands without bending the knees in the final position. Drop neck slowly and hold for some time breathing normally. Inhale slowly and come back to the original position.

37. Padmasana (Lotus Pose):

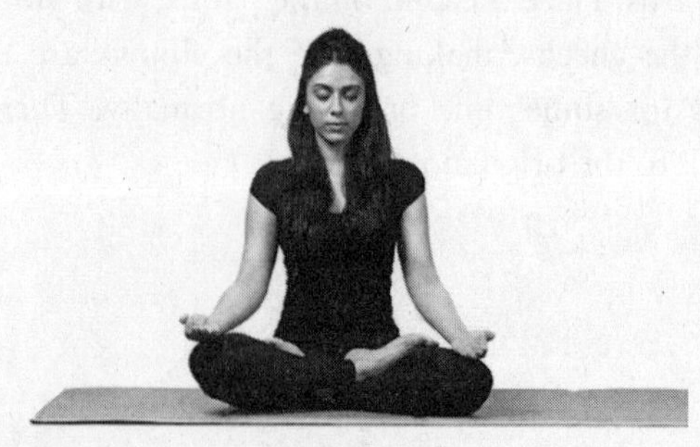

Sit on the floor and stretch the legs forward. Place the palms on the side of the body. Now, holding the sole of the right foot, place it on the left thigh and holding the sole of the left foot, place it on the right thigh. Keeping the back straight, place the palms on the knees in Gyan Mudra. Close your eyes slowly and focus on breathing normally. Hold for some time and come back slowly to the original position.

38. Parvatasana (Mountain Pose):

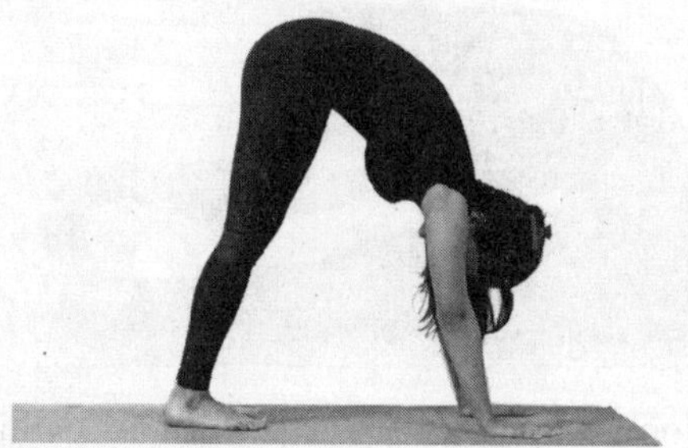

See Suryanamaskar.

39. Parvatasana in Padmasana (Mountain Pose in Lotus Seating):

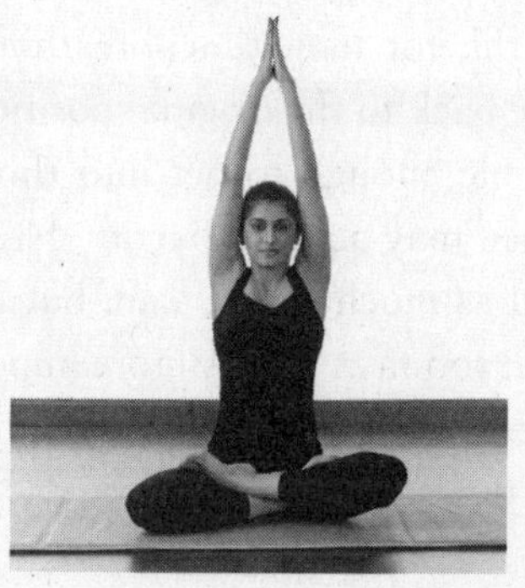

Sit straight in Padmasana with palms resting on the floor. Get the palms together, facing each other, in Namaskar Mudra close to the chest. Inhale slowly and raise your hands upwards and stretch your arms as much as you can without exerting pressure on the neck. Breathe normally and hold for some time. Slowly come back to the original position.

40. Paschimottanasana (Forward Bending):

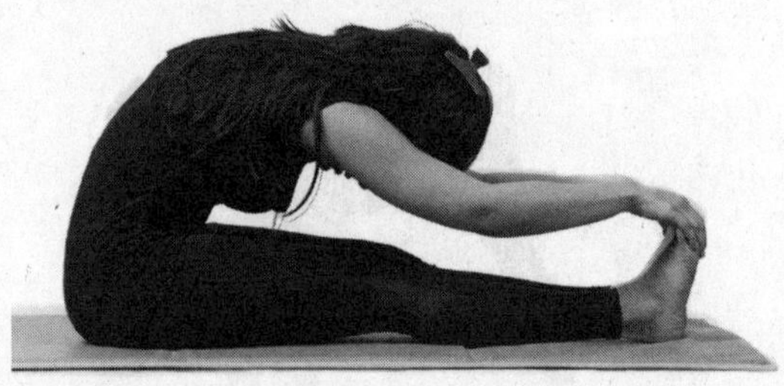

Sit on the floor, with your legs straight and palms on your thighs, keeping your heels on the floor. Inhale and take your hands upwards with your palms facing each other. Now bend forward and try to hold your foot with the help of your hands, without bending your knees. Keep bending forward as much as you can, while trying to touch your knees with your nose. Hold this for some time, breathing normally, and then slowly come back to the original position. Initially, one may not be flexible enough to get into this posture as the fat in the abdomen may act as a barrier. Nonetheless, at the initial stage bend as much as you can, but don't bend your knees. Don't do it too fast, as it is more important to remain in the bending posture for a longer duration than doing it more number of times.

41. Pawanmuktasana (Wind Relieving Pose):

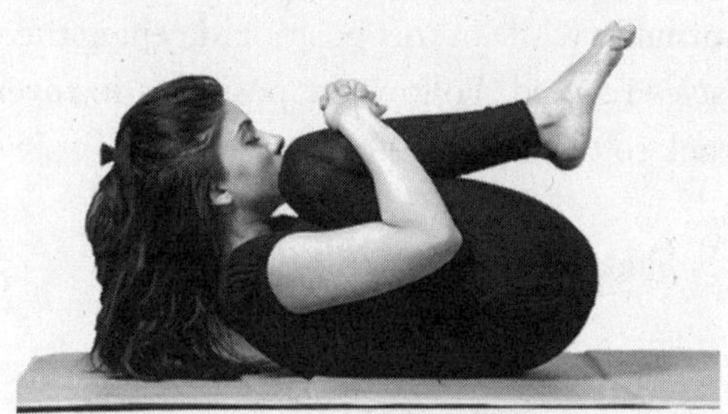

Lie on your back with your legs together, hands by the side, and palms resting on the floor. Slowly bend both knees together towards the chest. Hold your knees with your hands and pull well towards the chest. Raise your chin up between the knees, and hold for some time, breathing normally. Then come back to the original position.

42. Poorna Halasana (Plough Pose):

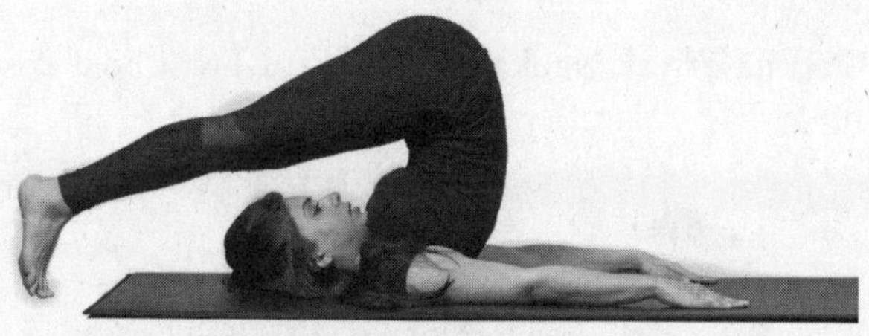

Lie on you back with feet together, hands by the side, and palms resting on the floor. Inhale, and then while exhaling raise both your legs up. With the help of your palms, raise your hips up and bring your toes above your head, without bending your knees. Now interlock your fingers with each other, stretch your arms together and hold the position. Breathe normally while in this position, keeping the neck and facial muscles relaxed. Follow the positions in reverse order to come back to the original position.

43. Poorna Shalabhasana (Locust Pose):

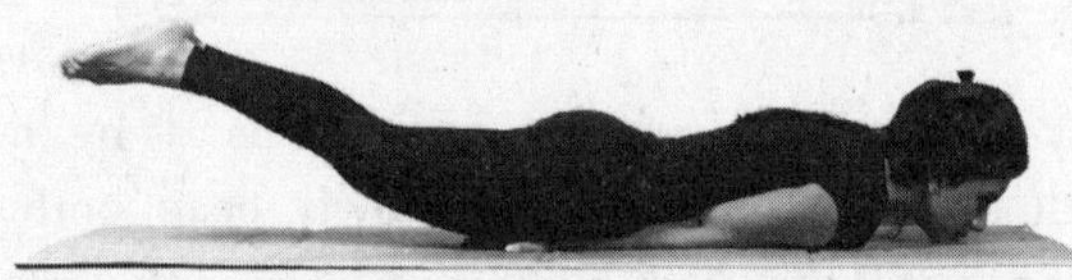

Lie in prone position. Bring the legs together, toes pointing outwards, hands by the side of the body, fists closed and take it under your thighs, and chin on the floor. While inhaling, raise both the legs slowly without bending at the knee. Do not tilt the pelvis. Hold this for some time breathing normally and come back down slowly.

44. Poorna Triyak Naukasana (Upward Twist Boat Pose):

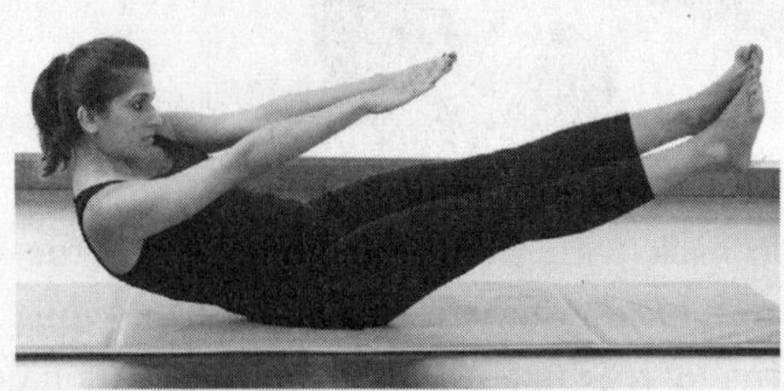

Lie on your back with your feet together and your palms resting on your thighs. Inhale slowly and raise both legs up. Then raise the upper body and hands upwards towards your toes. Now turn your full body towards the right side of your right hip. Hold for some time and come back to the original position. Repeat the same with the other side.

45. Push-ups (in Santolanasana):

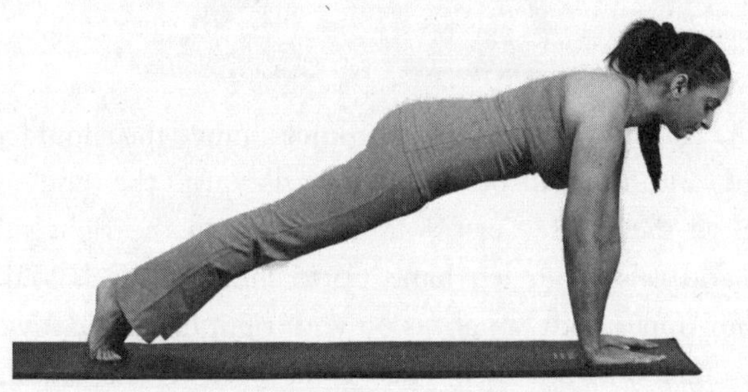

Sit in cat pose on the floor and take both your legs behind making sure your hands are aligned below your shoulder. The shoulders, back, AND hips should be in one straight line. Breathe normally when you're in this posture. While inhaling, bend your elbows as much as you can in this position and while exhaling push your palms, keeping your elbows straight. Keep repeating this movement. If you find it difficult then keep your knees on the floor and hip downwards with your body weight forward and do the same movement.

46. Santolanasana Variation 2 (With One Hand Upwards):

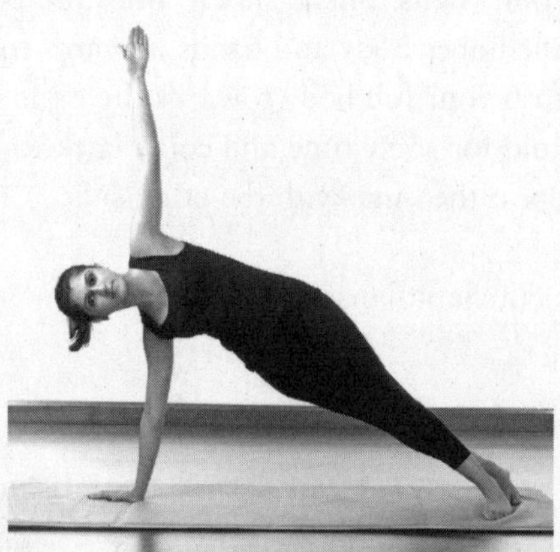

Sit in the cat pose, straighten your knees, move the shoulders forward and the buttocks downwards until the body is parallel to the floor. Turn your full body to the right side slowly and raise your left hand up to shoulder level. Make sure your upper body weight is on your right hand and lower body weight on both legs. Then come back to the original position. Repeat the same with the other side. Hold for some time, breathing normally.

47. Santolanasana Variation 3 (Hand Behind the Back):

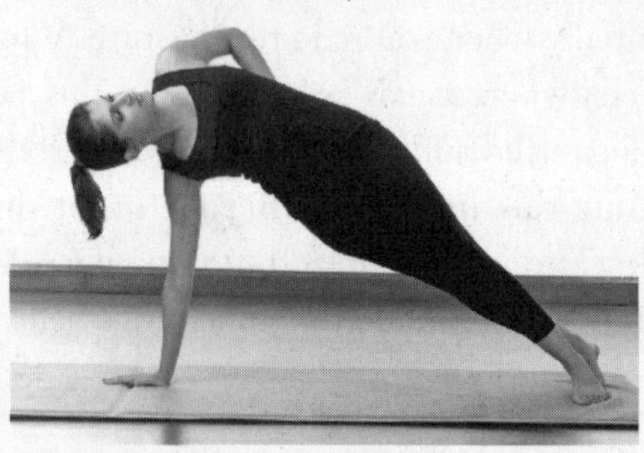

Sit in cat pose, straighten your knees, move the shoulders forward and the buttocks downwards until the body is straight like in position no. 5 of Suryanamaskar. Now turn the body to the right side and balance it on one hand taking the other hand behind the back and pushing the shoulder towards the ceiling. Hold for some time while breathing normally. Then slowly repeat with the other side.

48. Sarpasana (Serpentine Pose):

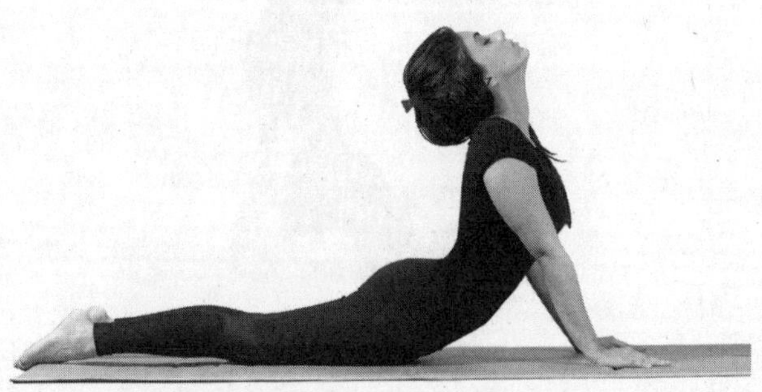

Lie on your stomach with your forehead touching the floor, hands by the side of your body, and palms by the side. Bend both your elbows slowly bringing your palms close to the chest, with elbows facing upwards close to your body. Inhale slowly raising your head, shoulders, chest, and stomach till your navel region, with the help of your hands. In the final position, hold for some time, breathing normally and then slowly come down to the original position.

49. Sarvangasana (Whole Body Pose):

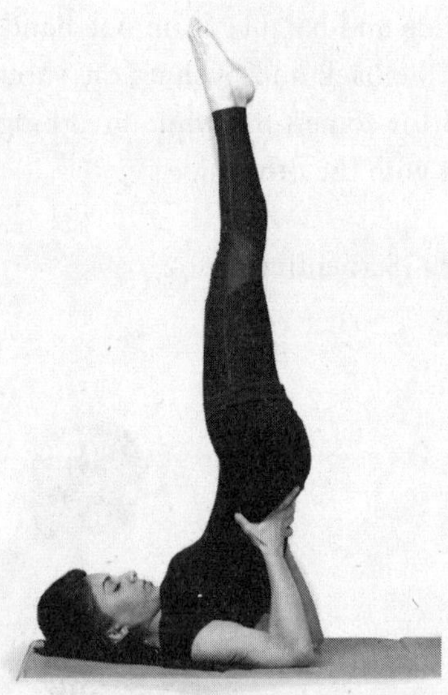

Lie down in the supine position with the legs together, hands by the side and palms facing the floor. Inhale slowly and while exhaling, raise both the legs together at a 90 degree angle to the floor. Now press the palms and bring the legs towards the head, so that the buttocks face upwards. Now bend the elbows and support the back with the palms. Then take the legs upwards till the legs, abdomen, and chest form a straight line. The chin should be placed against the jugular notch. Hold this for some time, breathing normally. While coming back to the original position first lower the buttocks, release the hands slowly and bring the legs down without raising the head.

50. Setubandhasana (The Closing Bridge Pose):

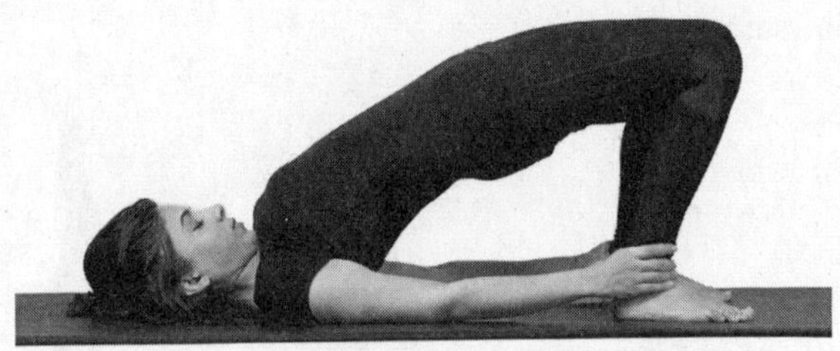

Lie on your back and bend your knees. Keep your feet close to your hips with hands by the side and palms resting on the floor. Inhale slowly and push the waist upwards as much as you can. Try gabbing your ankles without any pressure on your neck. Hold for some time while breathing normally.

51. Shavasana (The Resting Corpse Pose):

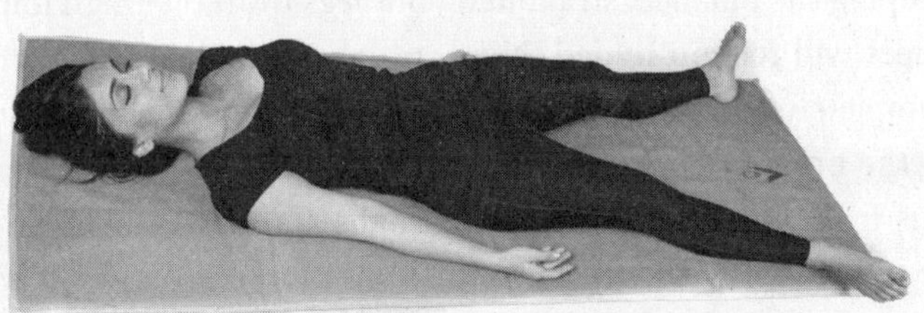

Lie down on the back with the legs together and hands by the side. Spread the legs apart slowly, keeping the heels inside and toes outside. Keep your hands away from the body, with the palms facing upwards. Close your eyes, loosen, and relax all the muscles in the body and focus on your normal and natural breathing.

52. Shirsasana

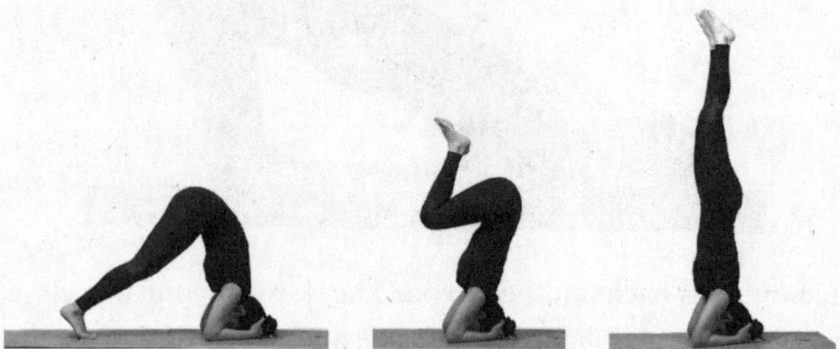

Sit on your soles and place your knees on the ground. Frame finger lock with both hands making a triangle from finger lock and elbows. Place it on the ground. Then bending forward, place the middle of your head on the ground near the finger lock. Now straighten your legs. Slowly bring the legs near your body. Soles will automatically leave the ground by practice and thighs and knees will touch the abdomen. Now keeping the balance, straighten your legs from the thigh joint; knees will remain folded. Now straighten the knees also and completely balance your body on your head. While returning to the original position, fold your knee first. Then fold your legs from the thighs and let the thighs and knees touch your abdomen. Now slowly place the soles on the ground. Slowly raise your head and sit on your soles.

53. Sidekick:

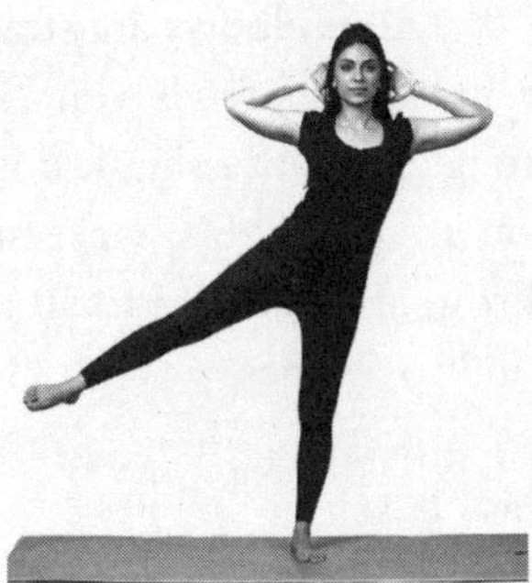

Stand straight with your feet shoulder width apart keeping your hands by the side of your body. Now interlock your fingers behind your head and slowly raise your right leg to the side focusing on your side muscles. Keep moving your leg sideways while exhaling. If you have a problem balancing, take the support of the wall. Repeat the same with the other side.

54. Simhasana (Lion Pose):

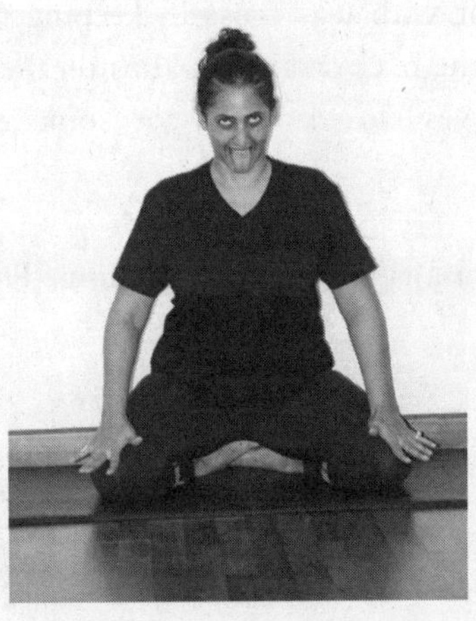

Sit in Vajrasana on your knees and place your palms on your knees, taking care that your elbows are straight. Now, inhale slowly and while exhaling stretch your facial muscles by pulling out your tongue and pressing it downwards towards the chin. While you are doing this, make sure that you look between your eyebrows. Hold for 15 to 20 seconds, breathing normally. Repeat it 3 to 5 times.

55. Sukhasana (Easy Pose):

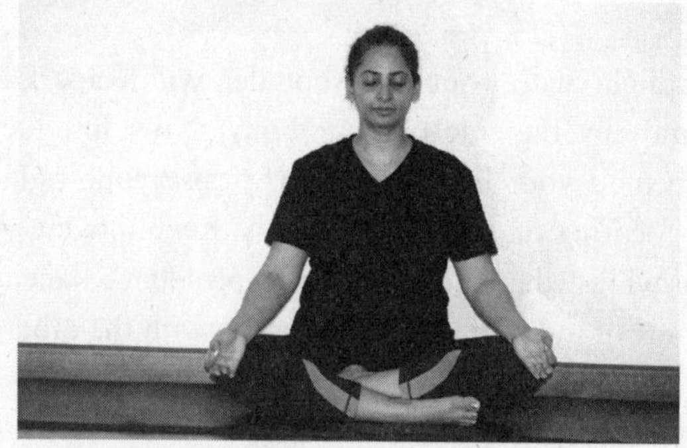

Sit on the floor with legs crossed, keeping the entire body relaxed. Keep the back straight, palms on the knees in Gyan Mudra, and eyes closed. Hold for some time, breathing normally.

56. Supta Vajrasana (Sleeping Adamantine Pose):

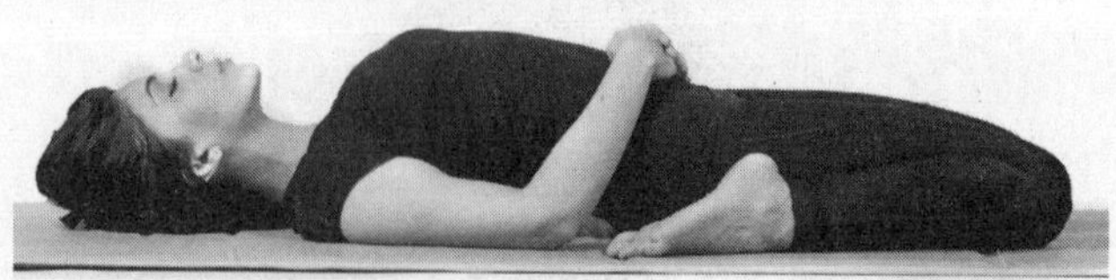

Sit straight in Vajrasana. Keep your feet apart on the floor. Lean backwards on your right and left elbows. Now try and bend your head and back towards the floor as much as you can till you are comfortable while stretching the abdomen. Keeping the hands on the thighs, hold for some time, breathing normally. Now with the help of the elbows slowly come back to the original position.

57. Tadasana (Mountain Pose):

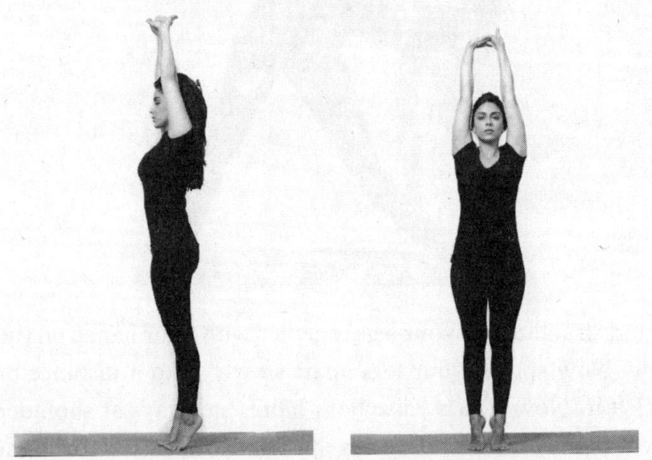

Stand straight with your feet shoulder width apart, and your hands to the side of your body. Inhale slowly raising your hands upwards with your palms facing each other. Stretch your entire body while standing on your toes. In the final position hold for some time, breathing normally. Come down to the original position slowly, while exhaling.

58. Trikonasana (Triangle Pose):

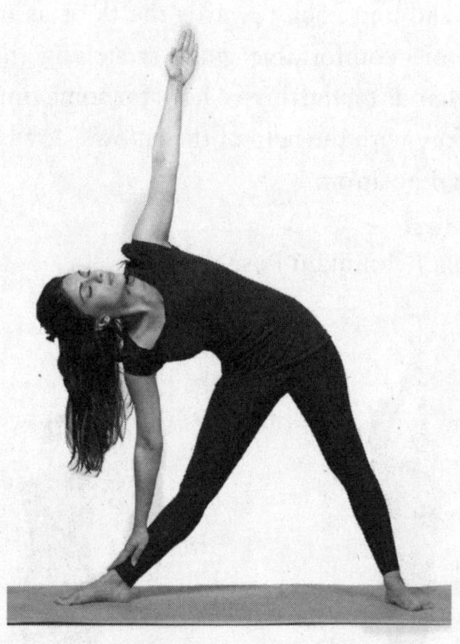

Stand straight with your legs together with your hands on the side. Now spread your legs apart slowly upto a distance of 2-3 feet. Now slowly raise both hands sideways at shoulder level with your palms facing down. Now turn your right toes out while exhaling and bend your upper body towards the right side touching the big toe of the right leg with right hand without bending the knees. Now raise your left hand up and look at your fingertips breathing normally. Hold this for some time and come back to the original position while inhaling.

59. Triyak Bhujangasana (Twisting Cobra Pose):

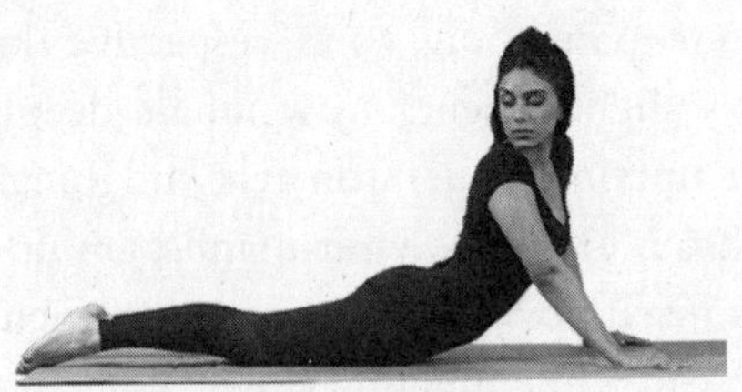

Lie in a prone position, with your legs together, toes together and pointing outwards, hands by the side of the body, palms facing upwards and forehead on the floor. Now bend hands from the elbows and place palms on the floor, near each side of the shoulder. The thumb should be under the armpit. Then inhale and raise the chin and turn the head backwards over the right shoulder as much as possible, and raise up to the navel. Hold for some time, breathing normally. Then while exhaling come downto the original position. Repeat the same with the left side.

60. Uddiyan Bandha (Upward Abdominal Lock):

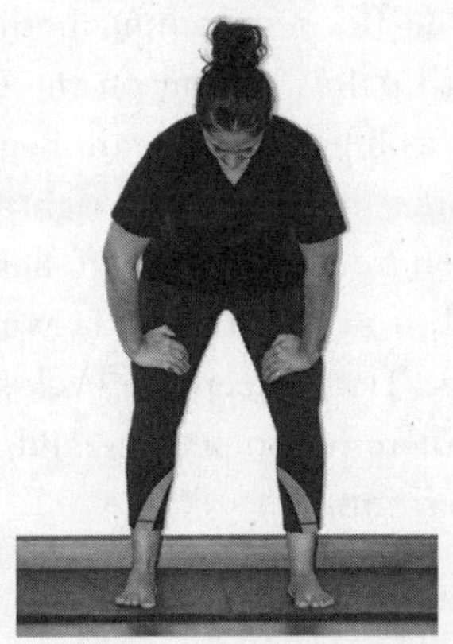

Stand straight with your feet shoulder width apart keeping your hands at the side of your body. Now bend your knees keeping your palms on your respective knees keeping your elbows slightly bent. Now inhale deeply and exhale forcefully emptying your stomach and lungs. Now hold your breath out and raise your diaphragm upwards, which will make a negative pressure on your stomach. Hold this as long as you can while inhaling slowly come back to normal position.

61. Ugrasana (Fierce or Powerful Pose):

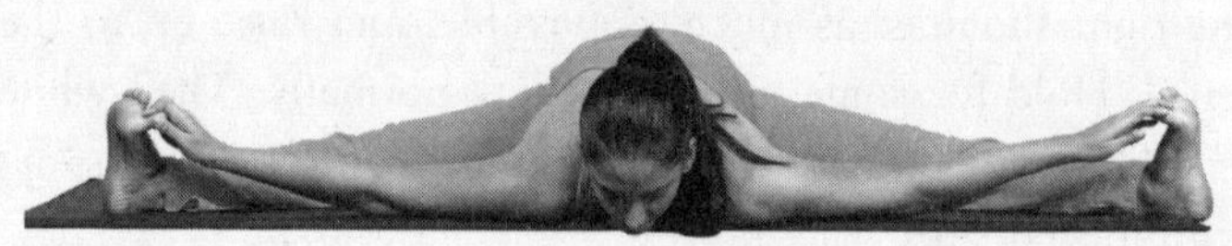

Sit straight on the floor stretching both legs together, in front of you, with palms resting on the floor. Now slowly spread your legs, as much as you can. Bend forward slightly and try to hold the big toe of the right leg with the right hand, and the left toe with the left hand. Now pull the toes inside slowly towards the body without bending the knees and elbows. Try to keep the back straight, breathing normally. Hold there for some time and slowly come back to the original position.

62. Upper Crunches:

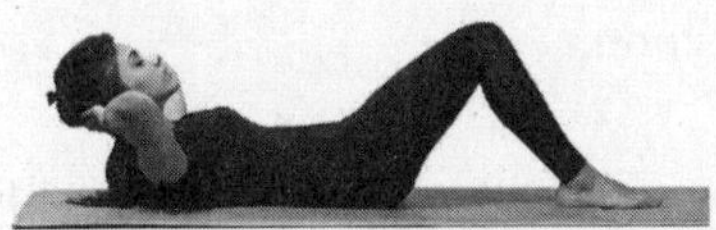

Lie on your back with your legs straighten in front and hands besides your body, palms facing downward. Slowly raise your hands behind your head and fold both your legs at the knee. Slowly keep lifting your head and crunching the upper abdominal muscles. As you come up exhale and inhale while going down.

63. Ushtrasana (Camel Pose):

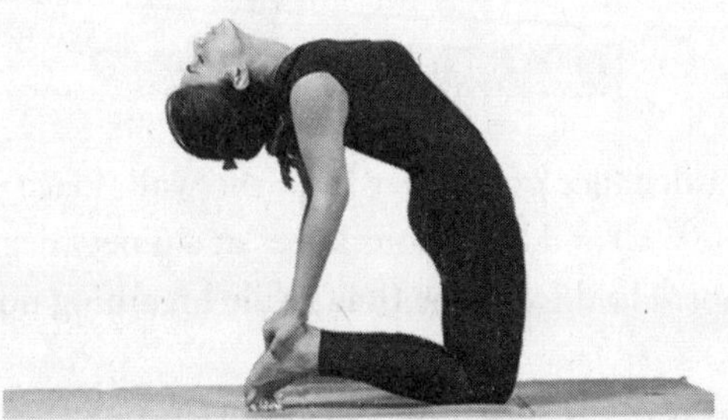

Sit straight in Vajrasana. Slowly stand on the knees keeping them shoulder width apart. Now slowly turn the upper body to the right side and try to catch the right heel with the right hand, and the left heel with the left hand while balancing the body. After holding the heels, inhale and push the waist forward and drop the neck back. Breath normally in the final position. Hold for some time. While exhaling come back to the normal position.

64. Utkatasana (Chair Pose Against the Wall):

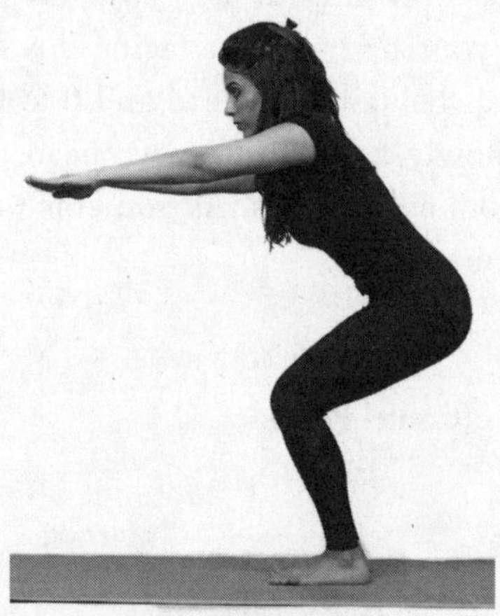

Stand at a distance of 1½ feet from the wall. Place your back against the wall and bend your knees at a ninety degrees angle to the floor. Hold for some time while breathing normally.

65. Utkatasana (Chair Pose) Levels 1 and 2:
Stand straight, feet together, palms by the side of the body. Keep your feet apart, almost as much as the width of your shoulders. Now bend your knees at 90 degrees to the floor

and slowly raise your hands in front of you to shoulder level.

Stay in this posture for some time and breathe normally. Slowly come back to the starting position. This is level 2. Level 1 is for beginners, wherein you bend your knees not up to 90 degrees to the floor but as much as you can comfortably.

66. Utkatasana (Chair Pose) Level 3:

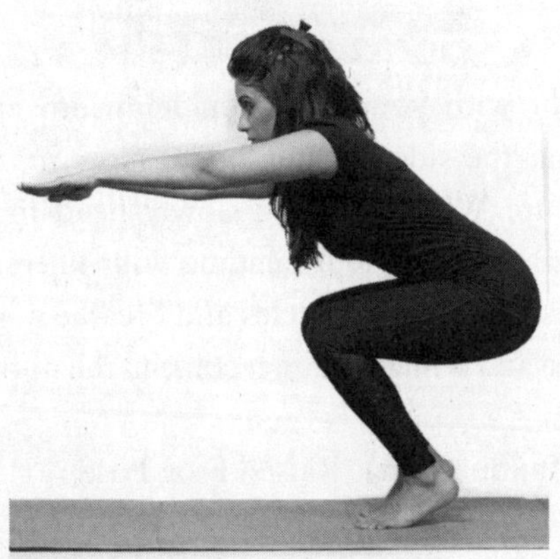

Stand straight, feet together, palms by the side of the body. Keep your feet apart, almost as much as the width of your shoulders. Now bend your knees at 90 degrees to the floor. Slowly raise your heels, balancing the body on your toes. Now raise your hands in front to shoulder level. Hold this posture, breathing normally.

67. Uttanasana (Intense Forward Bending):

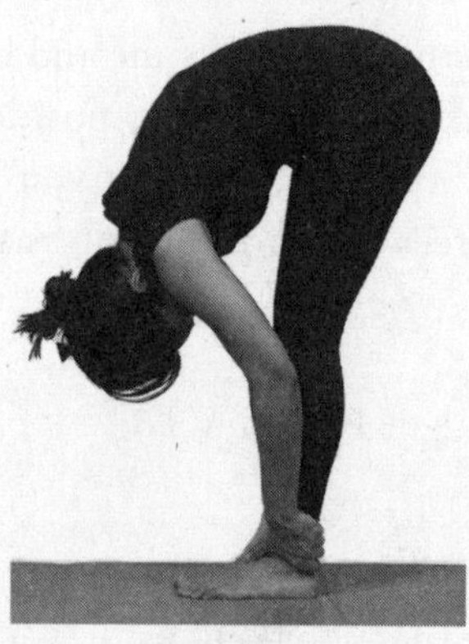

Stand straight with your feet shoulder width apart keeping your hands at the side of your body. Now inhale and raise both hands up. While exhaling slowly bend forward trying to catch your ankle without bending your knees. In the final position, relax your neck muscles and breathe normally. Hold for some time and while inhaling, come in the normal position.

68. Uttan Mandukasana (Raised Frog Pose):

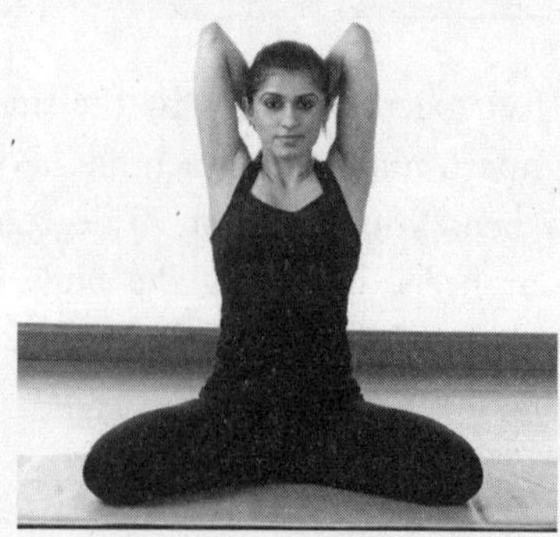

Sit in Vajrasana. Now spread both the knees and make sure the toes are touching each other, keeping the back straight. Bend the right hand backwards from above the right shoulder and place the palm below the left shoulder. Now, bending the left hand, place the palm on the right shoulder. Keeping the back and neck straight, breathe normally. Be in this position for some time. Come back slowly to the original position.

69. Vajrasana (Adamantine Pose):

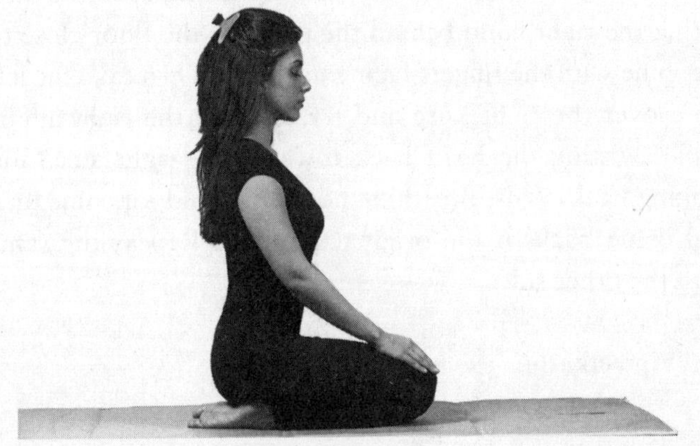

Sit with legs extended forward together, hands by the side of the body, and palms resting on the floor. Now bend the right leg at the knee and place the foot under the right buttock. Similarly, bend the left leg, and place it under the left buttock. Hands should be resting on the thighs with the back straight. Hold for some time then come back to the original position.

70. Vakrasana (Twisted Pose):

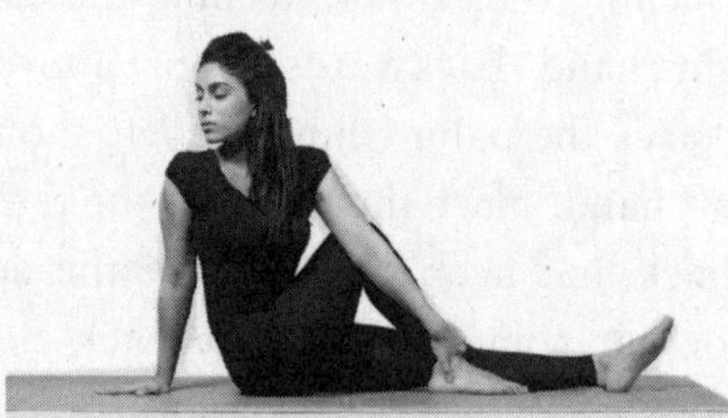

Sit straight on the floor, stretching the legs in front, hands by the side, and palms resting on the floor. Now slowly bend the right leg at the knee and place your right foot close to the left knee joint. With the right knee facing upwards now taking the right hand behind the palm on the floor close to the spine with the fingers facing upwards. Then take the left hand over the right knee and try to catch the right ankle, while twisting the head back towards the right side, and looking backwards. Breathing normally, hold for some time and come back to the original position. Repeat the same with the other side.

71. Vipreetkarni:

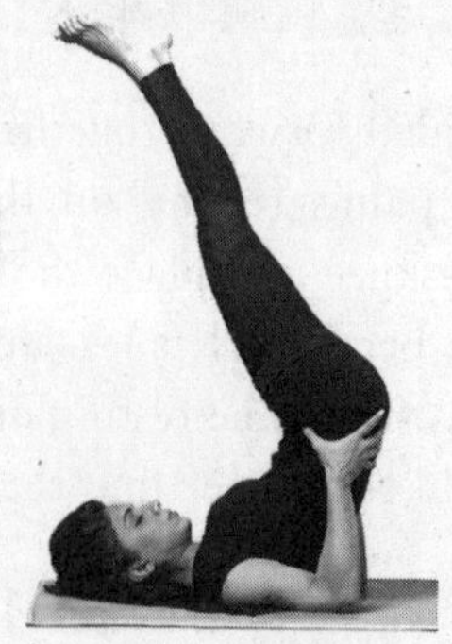

Put your feet together and hands by the sides with the palms resting on the floor. Now inhale slowly and raise both your legs up, 90 degrees to the floor. Then push your palms on the floor and raise your hips up. Hold your waist with your hands in the final position. Remember to keep your neck muscles relaxed and breathe normally. Stay in this position for 15 to 20 seconds, then come back slowly to the original position in a reverse manner. Follow it up with its counter pose Setubandhasana.

72. Virbhadrasana (Warrior Pose):

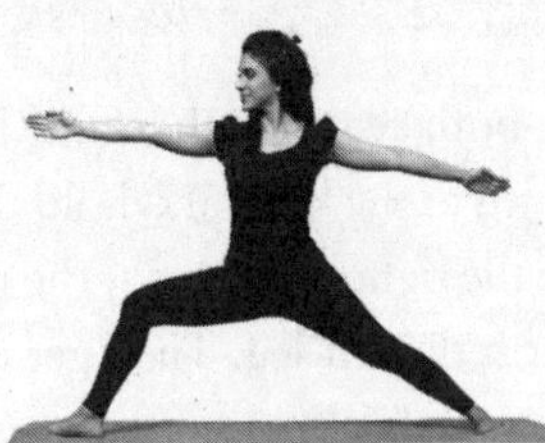

Stand straight with your feet shoulder width apart keeping your hands at the side of your body, now widen your legs apart 3-4 feet from the body. Now spread your arms sideways at shoulder level turn your right foot outwards. Bend your right knee 90 degrees from the floor and stretch your right arm towards your right side stretching your body as much as you can to the right side breathing normally. Do the same with the other side.

73. Vrikshasana (Tree Pose):

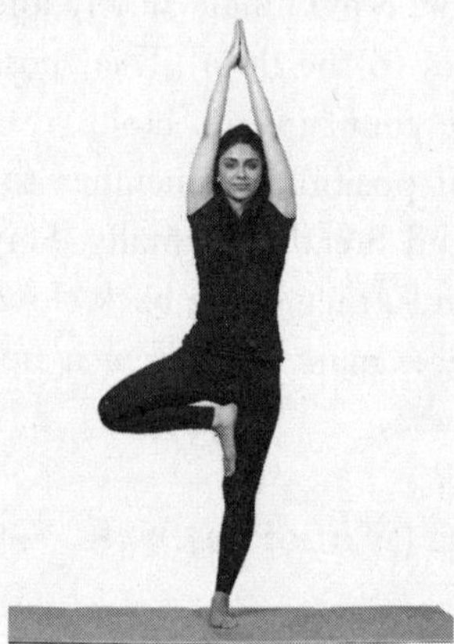

Stand straight with both feet together and hands by the side. Now bend the right leg at the knee and hold the right ankle with the right hand. Place the right heel tight at the pelvic region, while balancing the body on the left leg. Then get into the Namaskar Mudra with palms together, close to the chest. Balance this asana for some time, breathing normally. Come back slowly to the original position and repeat the same with the other leg.

74. Yoga Mudra:

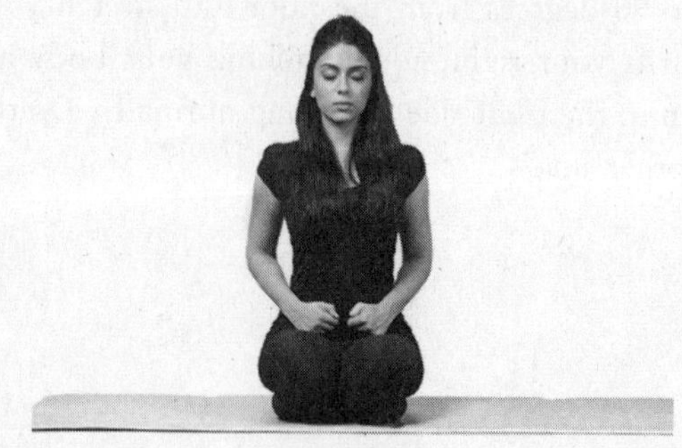

Sit in Vajrasana with your back straight and hands at the side of your body. Now close both your fist and put them on your thighs close to your navel region. Now inhale deeply. While exhaling, bend forward down touching your head on the floor and with your elbows relaxed. Hold this for some time breathing normally. While inhaling come back to the normal position.

This brings us to the end of Part one of the book. In this part I have tried to give you the practical information on the basics of yoga which you will find useful while understanding and doing the workouts in Part two. I have spent months designing the workouts for various issues that you will read about in the following chapters and I really wanted to include pictures and descriptions for all of them. So buckle up and let's get down to applying what we have learnt in the following chapters.

PART TWO

I AM A GIRL, NOT YET A WOMAN (15–25 YEARS)

Growing up is not easy but we all have to go through the grind sooner or later. From our parents' loving care we swiftly make our way to school, make friends, study for examinations, have fun and gradually step into teenage. Once you turn fifteen, and high school takes over, life seems to change completely. From a kid, you suddenly transform into a girl faced with lots of options and decisions. When I was growing up, I saw how my friends around me were opting for paths that their parents wanted them to follow. There was peer pressure and comparison between kids, and sadly a few of my friends could never follow their dreams. I too tried my hand at interior designing before I found my vocation in yoga. As you mature, your responsibilities increase and you venture out into the world. As you venture into adulthood, you start thinking about what you want to do for the rest of your life.

I feel 15–25 is a phase of transition—the formative period in every girl's life. It is also the best time to explore new horizons since a lot of opportunities open up before you. I remember how as a teenager I was a carefree soul who loved sports and having a good time. I was also creative which encouraged me to study interior design in college, and then my passion for fitness got me to learn yoga.

From a girl to a woman, adolescence to adulthood, the transformation is magical. You grow not just physically, but also emotionally and psychologically. Social interactions become a vital part of life as you make friends (real and virtual nowadays), develop your tastes, hobbies, likes and dislikes. This is the phase when you hone your personality and step out into the world. The primary focus zooms out from family and siblings, and zooms in to school, college, friends, career and new relationships. Let us talk more about this stage in our lives and understand what the important health concerns are during this time.

BEING A YOUNG ADULT

I meet a lot of young adults every day and know that being a young adult is quite challenging. It is a stage where your aim is to find your true self and fit in with others. As a young adult you develop critical thinking and discover newly found independence. With liberty also comes responsibility and you have to be sure not to misuse this freedom. I know a lot of you hate it when parents or teachers interfere in your 'personal life'. It is true that a girl goes through a lot while growing up. She has to deal with periods, peer pressure, sexuality, breast development, PMS, mood swings, stress, social life, and what not. But being a young adult isn't all that difficult either. This is also a time when you shape your career and future lives.

Nowadays a lot of girls start working early in life whether it is modelling, films or starting out their own ventures. There are actors like Alia Bhatt, Zoa Morani, Sonakshi Sinha who have started their careers early in life and are doing very well. I remember Sushmita Sen who became Miss India at the age of 19 and then went on to win the crown of Miss Universe. All of these lovely ladies have worked extremely hard to get where they are and also managed to look beautiful. Yoga changed Zoa Morani's life as she often says and made her focus better. It made her feel beautiful not only on the outside but also from within. However, I am not denying the changes and challenges of this age that we all have to deal with. Let us now try and understand a few important things that every girl should know.

PUBERTY

Puberty is one of the most significant stages of a girl's life. During this time we all undergo a lot of physical and emotional changes. Puberty paves the way for adulthood, sexual maturity and an awareness of being a woman. It is also the time when a woman's reproductive organs become functional and she starts getting her period.

The age at which a girl attains puberty is usually earlier than boys. Most girls reach this stage by the age of fifteen. If you are around that age you might as well ask yourself, 'Do I know why my body is experiencing so many changes?' 'Am I sexually aware?' I am quite sure many of you find it difficult to cope with hormonal fluctuations and hence do not understand the changes your body is going through. Some girls tend to get confused, and end up becoming shy and introverted. I really feel it is important for mothers, elders or schools to provide them with correct information about what is going on and that it is totally normal. Now let us try and understand what these fluctuations or changes mean.

Physical changes

Puberty in girls is marked by the production of sexual hormones, estrogen, progesterone, and small amounts of testosterone. The first sign of physical growth is through breast development. Also known as breast budding, this development is followed by other changes like growth of pubic hair, onset of the menstrual cycle commonly called periods, increase in weight and height, and also the widening of hips. All of you must have experienced your body's gradual transformation. I still remember meeting Mitali, a high school student, who seemed extremely upset about these changes. She couldn't understand why she had to go through all of this, have periods unlike the boys or why she had to wear a bra. I had to explain that it was a natural process which every girl goes through. All you need to know is how to deal with it without stressing about it.

Period is not just a punctuation mark

The first period or menarche normally begins anytime between 9 to 16 years. In the first year, periods are very light and may also be irregular. It is quite normal, so do not worry. It usually lasts for 3 to 7 days and the amount of blood flow varies from person to person. For some of you, it might be quite light while for others it might be heavy. As you grow up, gradually the amount of flow also increases. If you experience painful periods, or miss them for more than six months, I would advise you to go and get yourself checked by a gynaecologist. However, you should always remember that it is something really normal, part of growing up and that all women go through it.

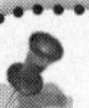

Let me give you a CLUE

Our world is full of apps but there are some which are really useful. Did you know there is an app called CLUE that helps predict your menstrual dates for up to 3 consecutive cycles? A lot of young people use it and it works wonders in predicting the right date for your menstrual cycle. So gone are the days of guessing dates and keeping fingers crossed. You could use technology to your benefit and be prepared early.

Why isn't PMS as cool as SMS?

PMS or premenstrual syndrome is a term which describes the physical and emotional fluctuations faced by a lot of women just before their periods. Almost 1 in every 3 women experiences PMS and it's more common than we might believe. It usually occurs a week or so before your menstrual cycles and can make you feel irritable and moody. Its symptoms increase at the onset and stop almost immediately after your periods end. Weight gain, sudden mood swings, nausea, fatigue, constipation, body ache, breast tenderness, and insomnia are some of the symptoms associated with it. Some women experience it more than the rest. Since it makes you grouchy and short-tempered, how do you deal with it? Following a balanced diet and sleeping well at night can actually help you keep PMS at bay. Moreover a cool, calm, composed mind can ward off all sorts of tensions.

School≠College

Time spent during school and college days are truly the most memorable. You have so much to learn, so much to explore. When I think about my school and college days I get nostalgic and wish those days could come back. This transition phase is marked by a lot of new experiences. School life is more disciplined and restricted while college life is marked by more freedom and life-altering decisions. These formative years form the foundation of who you are and will be. With new discoveries and technological advancements, life has changed tremendously. The kind of education I had might be totally different from what the kids learn nowadays. Knowledge is easily accessible and every person can now explore new vistas of learning. You just need to make learning more interesting, work hard and follow your dreams.

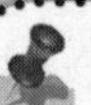

Useful Yoga Postures for Glowing Skin and Beauty

1. Jalneti Kriya: You could do it on alternate days for facial glow.
2. Trataka Kriya: Trataka Kriya is very good for the eyes. You can do it everyday for sparkling eyes.
3. Kapalabhati Kriya: This is very useful kriya for your skin. You should do it everyday for facial and internal glow.
4. Vipreetkarni: Vipreetkarni improves the blood circulation. You can do 3 to 5 rounds daily for good blood flow towards upper body.
5. Sarvangasana: Sarvangasana is also good for your skin and you could do 3 to 5 rounds for the unmistakable glow on your face.

(*Cont.*)

6. Matsyasana: This is a very useful exercise to improve your posture and overall appearance. You could do 3 to 5 rounds daily.
7. Shirsasana: This posture directs the flow of the blood towards the head. For best results do 2 rounds, each round being of 15 to 20 seconds in duration.
8. Shavasana: 5 minutes of Shavasana will make you feel and look peaceful and calm.

Note: For explanation please go to Chapter 6

Examination=Stress

Examination is common to both school as well as college. More and more students nowadays face exam stress. I feel sad when I see my 8-year-old niece worrying about her exams and not being able sleep or eat well. Yes, it is not only with older kids. Even younger children sometimes find it difficult to cope with the pressures of getting good grades and living up to their parents' expectations. So what is it you can do? Studying regularly rather than leaving everything for examination time is one of the solutions. Learn from your mistakes, talk to your parents and teachers about your weak areas, work on your style of studying, and be a little more proactive. These tiny steps can surely help you perform better and also look at examinations differently. Just try and work a little harder as well as smarter. If you are well prepared from the very beginning and plan well, stress will never affect you. Examination will always seem like a new challenge to analyse your skills. You could also try yoga and meditation to calm you down and help you focus better. To help you focus better you could try postures like Natarajasana,

Vrikshasana, and Garudasana. For meditation, I recommend Trataka Asana, sitting in Vajrasana, deep breathing observation, Bhramari, and Shavasana.

Am I a gizmo geek?

We are living in an age in which gadgets form a crucial part of life. One cannot even imagine leaving home without a mobile phone. Our lives are getting more and more dependent upon gadgets. Isn't it so? Priya, a 15-year-old girl I met in Pune, is addicted to her iPhone. So is Betsy. A 10-year-old, she says, she cannot live without her Xbox and spends several hours everyday glued to it.

Gizmos have become more or less a necessity for all of us. Virtual identities are part of our reality considering the amount of time we spend on the internet. You can't really think of life without Facebooking or texting, can you? Tweeting has made short conversations so interesting, hasn't it? From Rose Day to Propose Day, just drop an e-card and all is well. Every option is at your fingertips, be it buying clothes or ordering food from online menus. What if there was no TV or computer? How difficult would it be to live without such luxuries? Moreover, commercial competitiveness has given birth to a horde of options. You can find all sorts of gadgets in the market. Be it a smart phone or a palm top, everyone wants to possess the best gizmo. It has, in fact, become a status symbol for even kids.

Gizmos can be fun if used judiciously. If not, it can lead to problems like weak eyesight, hearing problems, stress, and BlackBerry thumb (caused due to continuously pressing of mobile phone buttons with the thumb). I feel it is good to be in tune with technology but it is equally important to enjoy the outdoor life, meet people, make real friends, and indulge in sports or exercise. How many of you are able to maintain this balance? A lot of us unfortunately can't and hence face several issues like teen obesity early in life. It's really sad how so many cases of teenagers being overweight is increasing in our country. I have seen the spurt in these cases myself in the past 5 years with worried parents bringing their kids to me to help them lose weight and stay fit. The reasons are varied from eating junk food, preferring outside food to fresh home-cooked fare, to lack of enough exercise, hormonal imbalance, and other health conditions related to lifestyle. To lose weight only exercise is not enough. You must also alter your diet and must consult a doctor if you have any health issues. As far as exercise is concerned, here is a workout I recommend for teenagers to get back into shape.

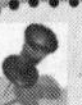

Workout for Teen Obesity

Total time: 1 hour 45 minutes

Best time to do it: Morning on an empty stomach or evening after a gap of 4-5 hours after your meal

1. Running on a treadmill at a speed of 6 to 8 km/h or outdoors, 1 hour
2. Rope skipping, 15 minutes
3. Warm up

a Upper body twist, 10 counts: Stand with legs slightly apart. Clasp the fingers behind the head. Press the elbows slightly back. During the whole exercise the soles of the feet remain flat

(*Cont.*)

on the floor, and upper body and head remain in a straight line. The legs remain straight during the twist.

- Inhale deeply.
- Exhaling, turn the upper body to the left.
- Inhaling, return to the centre.
- Exhaling, turn the upper body to the right.
- Inhaling, return to the centre.

b Arms stretching, 10 counts:

- Extend one hand down the centre of your back, fingers pointing downward.
- Use the other hand to grasp the elbow.
- Exhale slowly, pulling gently downward on your elbow, aiming to take your fingers along your spine.

c Shoulder rotation, 10 counts:

- Cross one arm horizontally over your chest, grasping it with either your hand or forearm, just above the elbow joint.
- Exhale, slowly pulling your upper arm in toward your chest.
- Aim to keep the hips and shoulders facing forward throughout the stretch.

d Neck stretch, 10 counts:

- Incline your head forward, but do not roll your head from side to side—this is dangerous. Instead, stretch your neck to the left, right, forward and back, but always return to the centre first!
- Tilt your head with ear toward shoulder, incline your head backward and roll your head from left to right, then right to left in a 30 degree motion.
- Be sure that while your head is tilted back, you keep your jaw relaxed and even let your mouth fall open just a bit.

e Forward stretch, 10 counts:

- Stand with your feet shoulder-width apart, one foot extended half a step forward.

(*Cont.*)

- Keeping the front leg straight, bend your rear leg, resting both hands on the bent thigh.
- Slowly exhale, aiming to tilt both buttocks upward, keeping the front leg straight, and both feet flat on the floor, pointing forward.
- Inhale slowly, and relax from this stretching exercise. Repeat the stretch again, this time beginning with the toes of the front foot raised toward the ceiling, but keeping the heel on the floor.

f Backward stretch, 10 counts:

- Stand with feet hip width apart and toes pointed forward. Reach both arms out in front of you and clasp your hands together.
- Now reach your arms out in front of you and turn your palms to face forward.
- Hold this stretch for about 30 seconds.

g Upward stretch, 10 counts:

- Extend both hands straight above your head, palms touching.
- Inhale, slowly pushing your hands upward, then backward, keeping your back straight.
- Exhale and relaxing from the stretch before you repeat.

h Side stretch, 10 counts:

- Stand with your feet together and your arms straight overhead. Clasp your hands together, with your fingers interlaced and pointer fingers extended.
- Inhale as you reach upward.
- Breathe out as you bend your upper body to the right. Take 5 slow breaths. Slowly return to the centre. Repeat on the left side.

i Leg stretch, 10 counts:

- Stand holding onto a secure object, or have one hand raised out to the side for balance.

(*Cont.*)

- Raise one heel up toward your buttocks, and grasp hold of your foot, with one hand.
- Inhale, slowly pulling your heel to your buttock while gradually pushing your pelvis forward.
- Aim to keep both knees together, having a slight bend in the supporting leg.

j Wrist rotation, 10 counts:

- Sit on the floor, legs stretched out straight before you, hands resting on your thighs.
- Close your eyes and breathe deeply for a few moments to prepare for the wrist rotation yoga exercises. Stretch your arms out straight in front of you, though be careful not to hyperextend at the elbows.
- With your arms stretched out straight, close your hands into fists, with your thumbs tucked inside. You need not clench. The fists should be loose and comfortable. slowly rotate your fists at the wrists—your right fist completing circles in a clockwise motion and your left fist completing circles in a counter clockwise motion. Complete 10 rotations.
- Switch the direction of each fist's rotation—your right fist now moving in a counter clockwise motion and your left fist now moving in a clockwise motion. Complete 10 rotations.

Take a break of 2 minutes after the warm up to begin with the exercises below:

4. Upper body crunches, 25 times, 4 rounds, with an interval of 10 seconds
5. Legs raises, 25 times, 4 rounds, with an interval of 10 seconds
6. Chakrasana, 2 rounds, with an interval of 10 seconds
7. Naukasana, 5 to10 rounds, with an interval of 5 seconds
8. Bhujangasana, 3 rounds, with an interval of 5 seconds
9. Kapalabhati, 200 to 500 times, 5 minutes
10. Relaxation in Shavasana, 5 minutes

THE WOES OF GROWING UP

With the advent of fast food and mall culture, life has changed dramatically. It is no longer cool to go out on picnics with family. In fact, children today want their own space and independence. They want to know everything, learn everything in a very short time. Such inquisitiveness has led to half-baked knowledge about most things. Google is the new agony aunt. Wiki Uncle has the solution to all the problems. Be it studies or sex, Harry Potter or porn, everything is available on the net. Are you too entangled in the web of World Wide Web? If yes, you need to know that data available on the net might be right but can also be misleading. You have to be careful about the source you refer to. It is a big world out there with thousands of answers to every single question. You yourself have to be on your guard.

JUVENILE DIABETES

As kids grow up, they often become more dependent on their friends and peers rather than family. Their choices are governed by not what they want to do but what everyone else is doing. At a very young age, they are exposed to tobacco, mall culture, alcohol, sex, fad diets, and drugs. Peer pressure can easily induce these behaviours and lead to addiction, teenage pregnancy, premarital sex, eating disorders, juvenile diabetes, teenage obesity, and other health problems.

I have particularly seen a lot more cases of juvenile diabetes in recent years. Meera Gupta,a 17-year-old girl, just passed her board examinations this year and has stepped into her college life. She used to feel weak and hungry at the same time and was experiencing nausea and frequent vomiting.

When she went to see the doctor, she was diagnosed with Juvenile Diabetes. There are more and more of such cases coming to light. There are several factors for it including genetic causes but it does help if you can maintain a healthy lifestyle, watch your weight, exercise regularly, and have a balanced diet. Here's a workout I recommend for Juvenile Diabetes.

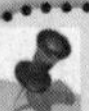

Workout for Juvenile Diabetes

Total time: 1 hour

Best time to do it: Morning on an empty stomach or evening after a gap of 4-5 hours after a meal

1. Padahastasana, 3 to 5 rounds, with an interval of 5 to 10 seconds
2. Trikonasana, 3 to 5 rounds, with an interval of 5 to 10 seconds
3. Vakrasana, 3 to 5 rounds, with an interval of 5 to 10 seconds
4. Paschimottanasana, 3 to 5 rounds, with an interval of 5 to 10 seconds (need to hold each posture for 10-15 seconds)
5. Pawanmuktasana, 3 to 5 rounds, with an interval of 5 to 10 seconds (need to hold each posture for 10-15 seconds)
6. Naukasana, 3 to 5 rounds, with an interval of 5 to 10 seconds (need to hold each posture for 10-15 seconds)
7. Bhujangasana, 3 to 5 rounds, with an interval of 5 to 10 seconds (need to hold each posture for 10-15 seconds)
8. Dhanurasana, 3 to 5 rounds, with an interval of 5 to 10 seconds (need to hold each posture for 10-15 seconds)
9. Kapalabhati, 100 to 200 times
10. Shavasana, 5 minutes for relaxation

OBESITY

Children, especially teenagers, may become rebellious and irritable in order to feel and look cool. With so many varieties of chips, biscuits, chocolates, and sodas available freely in the market it is no wonder that kids get into a wrong eating pattern and end up putting on a lot of weight. Moreover, as gadgets and games are taking over our lives, physical activity has considerably reduced leading to obesity among teenagers. Once you pile on several extra kilos it is very difficult to lose weight until you get serious and resolve to bring about a long term change in your lifestyle. Purva is a 24-year-old girl working at a leading hotel. During the last winter she let go of herself, partied a lot, attended several weddings, ate anything and everything without exercising and put on 9 kilos. She is now desperate to lose weight and get back into shape but is finding it extremely difficult to do it. So as they say, precaution is better than cure; one should always be on their guard. Do not get misguided by peers or adverts on TV. Think for your own good, your health, and your well being. Since I get a lot of queries about how to lose weight and deal with obesity in this age group, I am sharing with you two workouts to help you lose weight.

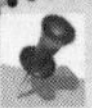

Workout if you are overweight by up to 8 kilos

Total time: 1 hour 30 minutes
Best time to do it: Morning on an empty stomach or evening after a gap of 4-5 hours after a meal

1. Walk for 45 minutes in the morning. You could walk on the treadmill or even brisk walk in the beach or garden

(*Cont.*)

2. Warmup, 5 minutes

a Upper body twist, 10 counts:

- Stand with legs slightly apart. Clasp the fingers behind the head. Press the elbows slightly back. During the whole exercise the soles of the feet remain flat on the floor and upper body and head remain in a straight line. The legs remain straight during the twist.
- Inhale deeply. Exhaling, turn the upper body to the left.
- Inhaling, return to the centre.
- Exhaling, turn the upper body to the right.
- Inhaling, return to the centre.

b Arms stretching, 10 counts:

- Extend one hand down the centre of your back, fingers pointing downward.
- Use the other hand to grasp the elbow.
- Exhale slowly, pulling gently downward on your elbow, aiming to take your fingers along your spine.

c Shoulder rotation, 10 counts:

- Cross one arm horizontally over your chest, grasping it with either your hand or forearm, just above the elbow joint.
- Exhale, slowly pulling your upper arm in toward your chest.
- Aim to keep the hips and shoulders facing forward throughout the stretch.

d Neck stretch, 10 counts:

- Incline your head forward, but do not roll your head from side to side—this is dangerous. Instead, stretch your neck to the left, right, forward and back, but always return to the centre first!

(*Cont.*)

- Tilt your head with ear toward shoulder, incline your head backward and roll your head from left to right, then right to left in a 30 degree motion.
- Be sure that while your head is tilted back, you keep your jaw relaxed and even let your mouth fall open just a bit.

e Forward stretch, 10 counts:

- Stand with your feet shoulder-width apart, one foot extended half a step forward.
- Keeping the front leg straight, bend your rear leg, resting both hands on the bent thigh.
- Slowly exhale, aiming to tilt both buttocks upward, keeping the front leg straight, and both feet flat on the floor, pointing forward.
- Inhale slowly, and relax from this stretching exercise. Repeat the stretch again, this time beginning with the toes of the front foot raised toward the ceiling, but keeping the heel on the floor.

f Backward stretch, 10 counts:

- Stand with feet hip-width apart and toes pointed forward. Reach both arms out in front of you and clasp your hands together.
- Now reach your arms out in front of you and turn your palms to face forward. Hold this stretch for about 30 seconds.

g Upward stretch, 10 counts:

- Extend both hands straight above your head, palms touching.
- Inhale, slowly pushing your hands upward, then backward, keeping your back straight.
- Exhale and relaxing from the stretch before you repeat.

(*Cont.*)

h Side stretch, 10 counts:

- Stand with your feet together and your arms straight overhead. Clasp your hands together, with your fingers interlaced and pointer fingers extended.
- Inhale as you reach upward. Breathe out as you bend your upper body to the right. Take five slow breaths. Slowly return to the centre. Repeat on the left side.

i Leg stretch, 10 counts:

- Stand holding onto a secure object, or have one hand raised out to the side for balance.
- Raise one heel up toward your buttocks, and grasp hold of your foot, with one hand.
- Inhale, slowly pulling your heel to your buttock while gradually pushing your pelvis forward.
- Aim to keep both knees together, having a slight bend in the supporting leg.

j Wrist rotation, 10 counts:

- Sit on the floor, legs stretched out straight before you, hands resting on your thighs. Close your eyes and breathe deeply for a few moments to prepare for the wrist rotation yoga exercises.
- Stretch your arms out straight in front of you, though be careful not to hyperextend at the elbows.
- With your arms stretched out straight, close your hands into fists, with your thumbs tucked inside. You need not clench. The fists should be loose and comfortable.
- Slowly rotate your fists at the wrists—your right fist completing circles in a clockwise motion and your left fist completing circles in a counter clockwise motion.

(*Cont.*)

- Complete 10 rotations. Switch the direction of each fist's rotation—your right fist now moving in a counter clockwise motion and your left fist now moving in a clockwise motion. Complete 10 rotations.

3. Front kicks, 50 each with both legs, 2 rounds
4. Sit ups, 25 times, 2 rounds
5. Suryanamaskar, 15 times, holding each posture for 5 seconds
6. Shavasana, 5 minutes, for relaxation

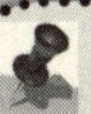

Workout if you are overweight by more than 8 kilos

Total time: 1 hour 50 minutes

Best time to do it: Morning before you start your day on an empty stomach

1. Alternate between walking and running for 45 minutes. Walk for 4 minutes at 6 km/h then run for 2 minutes at 8 km/h
2. Warm up

a Upper body twist, 10 counts:

- Stand with legs slightly apart. Clasp the fingers behind the head. Press the elbows slightly back. During the whole exercise the soles of the feet remain flat on the floor and upper body and head remain in a straight line. The legs remain straight during the twist.
- Inhale deeply.
- Exhaling, turn the upper body to the left.
- Inhaling, return to the centre.
- Exhaling, turn the upper body to the right.
- Inhaling, return to the centre.

(*Cont.*)

b Arms stretching, 10 counts:

- Extend one hand down the centre of your back, fingers pointing downward.
- Use the other hand to grasp the elbow.
- Exhale slowly, pulling gently downward on your elbow, aiming to take your fingers along your spine.

c Shoulder rotation, 10 counts:

- Cross one arm horizontally over your chest, grasping it with either your hand or forearm, just above the elbow joint.
- Exhale, slowly pulling your upper arm in toward your chest.
- Aim to keep the hips and shoulders facing forward throughout the stretch.

d Neck stretch, 10 counts:

- Incline your head forward, but do not roll your head from side to side—this is dangerous. Instead, stretch your neck to the left, right, forward and back, but always return to the centre first!
- Tilt your head with ear toward shoulder, incline your head backward and roll your head from left to right, then right to left in a 30 degree motion.
- Be sure that while your head is tilted back, you keep your jaw relaxed and even let your mouth fall open just a bit.

e Forward stretch, 10 counts:

- Stand with your feet shoulder-width apart, one foot extended half a step forward.
- Keeping the front leg straight, bend your rear leg, resting both hands on the bent thigh.
- Slowly exhale, aiming to tilt both buttocks upward, keeping the front leg straight, and both feet flat on the floor, pointing forward.

(*Cont.*)

- Inhale slowly, and relax from this stretching exercise. Repeat the stretch again, this time beginning with the toes of the front foot raised toward the ceiling, but keeping the heel on the floor.

f Backward stretch, 10 counts:

- Stand with feet hip-width apart and toes pointed forward. Reach both arms out in front of you and clasp your hands together.
- Now reach your arms out in front of you and turn your palms to face forward. Hold this stretch for about 30 seconds.

g Upward stretch, 10 counts:

- Extend both hands straight above your head, palms touching.
- Inhale, slowly pushing your hands upward, then backward, keeping your back straight.
- Exhale and relax from the stretch before you repeat.

h Side stretch, 10 counts:

- Stand with your feet together and your arms straight overhead. Clasp your hands together, with your fingers interlaced and pointer fingers extended.
- Inhale as you reach upward. Breathe out as you bend your upper body to the right.
- Take 5 slow breaths. Slowly return to the centre. Repeat on the left side.

i Leg stretch, 10 counts:

- Stand holding onto a secure object, or have one hand raised out to the side for balance.
- Raise one heel up toward your buttocks, and grasp hold of your foot, with one hand.

(*Cont.*)

- Inhale, slowly pulling your heel to your buttock while gradually pushing your pelvis forward.
- Aim to keep both knees together, having a slight bend in the supporting leg.

j Wrist rotation, 10 counts:

- Sit on the floor, legs stretched out straight before you, hands resting on your thighs.
- Close your eyes and breathe deeply for a few moments to prepare for the wrist rotation yoga exercises.
- Stretch your arms out straight in front of you, though be careful not to hyperextend at the elbows.
- With your arms stretched out straight, close your hands into fists, with your thumbs tucked inside. You need not clench. The fists should be loose and comfortable. slowly rotate your fists at the wrists—your right fist completing circles in a clockwise motion and your left fist completing circles in a counter clockwise motion.
- Complete 10 rotations. Switch the direction of each fist's rotation—your right fist now moving in a counter clockwise motion and your left fist now moving in a clockwise motion. Complete 10 rotations.

3. Front kicks, 50-50 with each leg, 2 rounds
4. Side kicks, 50-50 on each side, 2 rounds
5. Suryanamaskars, 25 times, slowly
6. Naukasana, 5 rounds, each round at an interval of 5 seconds. Hold each posture for 15 seconds
7. Setubandhasana, 2 rounds. Hold each posture for 15 seconds
8. Kapalabhati, 200 times
9. Shavasana, 5 minutes, for relaxation

If you ask me, this stage in a woman's life is the most precious. I still get nostalgic when I think about my college days, and those carefree, fun moments spent with friends in the college canteen. How I wish it could last forever! But life goes on and keeps on teaching us practical lessons, bringing with it new adventures and fresh set of experiences. The important thing is to value what we have, respect our body and take care of it as this is what will come in handy later in life.

MIDLIFE? NOT YET (25–35 YEARS)

Real life begins after twenty-five. Isn't it true? Till twenty-five, you are still learning, growing up, and slowly attaining maturity. Once you cross life's silver jubilee, the silver lining associated with childhood and adolescence slowly fades away. So what happens next? Your priorities change. Studies more or less take a back seat, and work life, career, love life, marriage, and household chores take precedence.

Unlike a few decades back, most women nowadays get married in their late twenties or even later in their thirties. After marriage, life takes a U-turn for most of us and you enter a totally new stage of your life. With marriage comes additional responsibilities. You have to take care of your home, husband, children, family, etc., besides your work and friends. You are no longer a free bird. You switch over to so many different roles: one moment you are a wife and the very next moment you have to be a mother or a daughter-in-law. There are many more people in your life; you have to remember so many birthdays and anniversaries, and simultaneously juggle everything, with a smile.

Wasn't life simpler and more carefree before getting married? As a single woman you never had to bother about relatives, friends, and family. But now you have two sets of families to manage, two sets of responsibilities. I remember when I was single how I could make a sudden plan to go on a holiday with my friends, go out to watch a late night film after work or come back home whenever I liked but after getting married and being a mother of a naughty 4-year-old those days seem a distant dream. However, it is best not to lose yourself in this transition. No matter how much time you spend on family and friends, you need to take out time for yourself and your health. You need to understand that your body needs rest and exercise. In fact, if you are healthy and fit you will most likely be happier and that will reflect in everything you do.

In light of all of these changes and important milestones in our lives, 25-35 I feel is the most important phase in your life. It is the time when you are at the crossroads of self-evaluation and decision making. The choices you make at this time decide your future whether it is to do with your life, relationships, or your body. Your decisions also establish who you are and what you want from your life. The path you tread on during this time is what eventually determines your destiny. You can either make it or break it both in terms of your career and your health. So we all should be careful and think hard before making our choices.

VISTAS OF LIFE

Why am I talking about career, work, love or marriage here? The answer is simple. Our mind and body are connected and have to be in sync for us to enjoy good health. Tension, unhappiness, and stress are the main causes of lifestyle diseases today. Obesity, diabetes, heart issues, PCOD, you name it. These are caused not only by our eating and exercise habits but also due to our mental condition. It is therefore extremely important to understand the important stages in our life and how it can affect the way we look and feel.

CAREER

Career for most women is one of the most important aspects of life today. Unlike before, women want to work and be independent. Being financially secure is crucial to most of us. We want to take charge of our lives and no longer depend on others for our needs. As such, setting up a career of your choice is one of the most important aspects of life.

If you do not enjoy your work, you'll never really be satisfied. Work on your weak areas and hone your skills. As a teenager and young adult you can try exploring options for yourself. After college, I got interested in interior design and did a course to get trained in it but eventually I found my calling in yoga. Like me, your preference should purely depend upon what you really want to do in life. Take suggestions and listen to the advice of people you look up to but do not let anyone else govern your choice. I still remember how Meenal cribbed about her job every other day. She wanted to pursue HR but due to family pressure she had to opt for Marketing. If only she had given it a thought and listened to what her heart and mind said, things wouldn't have been so disappointing. My only suggestion would be to look at the pros and cons of career options. There's no point cribbing later.

WORK

Okay, so you are a busy working woman who spends almost half a day in office. Your work shapes not just your personality but also your perspective towards life, family, health and so on. If you love your work, life would seem smooth and exciting. If not it would surely be monotonous and dull. Nine to five jobs, office politics, managing home and work life, and desk jobs can not only be tiring but also quite distressing. Seema Gulati is a 29-year-old PR executive. She is a workaholic and loves meeting people, talking and travelling but that means she is often out with her clients, entertaining them and thinking of new ideas. While Seema loves her job she is also a mother of a school going kid and often feels guilty about not devoting enough time to her family. Are you going through a similar dilemma? So how does one deal with it?

Work stress and balancing your personal and professional life can be easy if you know how to manage time. Being proactive can actually help you meet deadlines in time. Keeping your cool is equally important. Be patient and never let anger affect you. In terms of healthy habits at work, eat at regular intervals, avoid eating foods that are too oily or spicy, take the stairs to your office, play any one sport you like, and practice pranayam and meditation every morning. And yes, don't forget to drink lots of water. The benefits of drinking 4-6 litres of water everyday are immense. It is especially important for you if you want to look like a goddess and have a glowing and blemish free skin. I feel, since water is mostly free, it is really underrated but remember it can be your secret weapon. Here are a few asanas you can try to stay away from office stress.

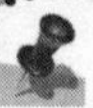

Yoga for office

Total time: 15 minutes

Best time to do it: You could do these anytime in office before meals. All these asanas can be done sitting on a chair

1. Brahma Mudra: 2 rounds
2. Parvatasana: 15 seconds, 2 rounds
3. Ardha gomukhasana: 15 seconds, 2 rounds
4. Vakrasana: 15 seconds on each side, 2 rounds
5. Paschimottanasana: 15 seconds, 2 rounds
6. Bhramari: 5 rounds
7. Om chanting with eyes closed, 3 rounds

PCOS Alert

Maya Gupta, 33, is a successful journalist. Her job involves long work hours, reporting, irregular meal times, and late nights. Her normal sleep time is around 1 am. Recently, she was diagnosed with PCOS (Poly Cystic Ovarian Syndrome) which has become an extremely common condition among women in India. PCOS is a common endocrine disorder affecting women mainly in their reproductive age. Few decades back, no one would have even heard of this in India but believe me it is now common especially in the metros and bigger cities. About 2-25 percent of women in India below the age of 45 have been found to be suffering from PCOS and the numbers are increasing every year. What can you do to prevent PCOS? Can yoga help? Here's a workout that you can do to deal with PCOS.

Yoga for PCOS

Total time: 1 hour

Best time to do it: Morning on an empty stomach or evening after a gap of 4-5 hours after your meal

1. Tadasnana: Hold for 15 seconds, 2 rounds
2. Supta Vajrasana: Hold for 15 seconds, 2 rounds
3. Ushtrasana: Hold for 15 seconds, 2 rounds
4. Yogmudra: Hold for 15 seconds, 2 rounds
5. Naukasana: Hold for 15 seconds, 2 rounds
6. Chakrasana: Hold for 15 seconds, 2 rounds
7. Counterpose Paschimottanasana: 1 time
8. Sarvangasana: 15 seconds, 1 round
9. Halasana: 15 seconds, 1 round
10. Counterpose Matsyasana: 15 seconds, 1 round
11. Sheetali Pranayam or Chandrabhedan Pranayam: 10 rounds each
12. Mooldhara Chakra activation

LOVE AND RELATIONSHIPS

Relationships are complicated, difficult to sustain and often end up in heartbreaks yet they govern our lives. Love evokes different emotions in different women but one thing is common—it makes you feel special. It makes you feel on top of the world, virtually like a goddess. No wonder we are ready to go to lengths to work hard and look good. I am sure most of you have experienced this feeling. When I fell in love with Manish, I felt as if I found a new meaning to my life. I was happy, laughing more than normal, and almost dreamy at times. More importantly, I wanted to look and feel beautiful all the time. Being at your optimal weight is definitely a good way to look good and fit into those lovely outfits to impress your partner. In case you are overweight and struggling to shed off some kilos, you can follow the below workout. The first routine is for those of you who are upto 8 kilos overweight while the second workout is for losing more than 8 kilos.

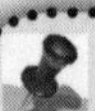

Workout for Obesity

Total time: 1 hour 15 minutes

Best time to do it: Morning on an empty stomach or evening after a gap of 4-5 hours after your meal

Upto 8 kilos

45 minutes walking, running or treadmill

Warm up for 5 minutes

Sit ups 30 times + front kicks 15 times + lunges 15 times each leg + push ups 15-20 times + 5 Suryanamaskars: 1 round; do 5 rounds

Kapalabhati-250 times

Shavasana-2 minutes

More than 8 Kilos

40-60 minutes cardio workout

Warm up 5 minutes

50-50 kicks against the wall, each leg

50-50 side kicks against the wall, each leg

10 sit ups + 2 Suryanamaskars, 5 rounds

Crunches upper body 25 times, 4 rounds

Leg raises lower body 25 times, 4 rounds

End with Setubandhasana or Chakrasana 1 time

Counterpose is Pawanmuktasana 3 times

Kapalabhati 250 times, 2 rounds

Love is an important ingredient of life, be it before marriage or after marriage. Whether your love is fulfilled or unfulfilled, till the time it lasts it makes you feel great. From adolescence, teenage to adulthood, we experience different kinds of love. Each experience teaches us something and helps us evolve into what we are today. A lot of women undergo stress due to break ups, divorce, fights, and arguments.

Rachna Sethi, 27, an IT professional was quite depressed when she met me last year. She had recently broken up with her boyfriend which had left her completely shattered. She would keep crying every now and then. I suggested she try out a yoga class. Slowly with time, things began to look up. She was not only looking hotter than before but she made new friends in her class. It really helped her self esteem and got her back on track. Now she is dating somebody else and is happier than before.

MARRIAGE

Marriage is probably the most important decision in a woman's life. You can find the middle ground on a lot of things but not your spouse, since such a compromise can be devastating. Before you take a step ahead, pause for a moment and ask yourself, is this what I really want to do? Am I getting married under any kind of pressure? Is this the person I truly love? Your fate is literally in your hands. Nobody is going to decide what you want in life. You need to be sure of your decision. Love marriage or arranged marriage, as long as you are happy and satisfied; nothing else really matters.

Smita Gupta and Rahul Singh met at their workplace and fell in love. At that time, Smita was only 23 and Rahul was 29. They got married within the next 3 months and they were happy for the first few months. However, within a year cracks seemed to appear in their marriage. Whether it is a love or an arranged marriage, do not take any decision in haste. If arranged marriage is your choice, do think about your preferences, your likes and dislikes too. Do not go for it blindly or without thinking.

Doesn't life change after marriage? Most of us in India put on weight after getting married. Mala Arora was 26 when she got married. Life was beautiful after marriage but the constant socializing and family dinners left a mark. She was not exercising and just going with the flow, enjoying the changes in her life. No wonder, from 56 kilos she was close to 70 kilos within a year. She is now struggling to lose all the extra kilos. This would probably be the story of so many newly married women in India. Before you can celebrate your first anniversary you start looking very different.

One of the most crucial periods when people put on weight is during their honeymoons. Honeymoon for most of us is the most cherished part of getting married. It marks the beginning of married life and also annoying weight gain. Since your hormones undergo a lot of changes, due to the changed environment, lifestyle, and sexual habits, your body too transforms accordingly. So are you too experiencing unwanted and sudden weight gain? You can blame it on the hormones but they are only partly responsible. The biggest culprit is lifestyle changes that occur post marriage. Living together with a man changes a woman's eating habits. On your honeymoon you eat out and enjoy lavish meals. When Pragya Thakur, 27, got married, she began to bulk up immediately. After gaining 5 kilos, she realized that her husband's snacking habits had somehow become hers too. She was nibbling on something or the other most of the time and had gained a lot of fat. These changes are common and happen with most women. So what can you do to keep your health on track and continue to look good? The most important thing is to keep track of your weight on a monthly basis and buy a weighing machine. Take you weight regularly and keep a monthly calendar so that you don't get a shock after 6 months or a year when it is already too late. Here's a workout to knock off those nagging post honeymoon kilos.

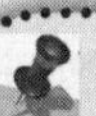

Workout for post honeymoon weight

Total time: 1 hour 15 minutes
Best time to do it: Morning on an empty stomach or evening after a gap of 4-5 hours after your meal

30 minutes running walking or treadmill
Suryanamaskars 25 times, 2 rounds
Upper body crunches 25 times, 5 rounds
Lower body crunches 25 times, 5 rounds
Naukasana 15 seconds 5 rounds
After each round you need to do Setubandhasana (for beginners) or Chakrasana (advanced level)
Kati Chakrasana 1 time each side
Kapalabhati 250 times, 2 rounds

PREGNANCY

During the twenties and thirties, there is another life transforming change that most women experience, the miracle of giving birth. Having a child is a wonderful experience and unforgettable. Becoming a mother is one of the most beautiful experiences and I can vouch for it. I got pregnant when I was almost 35 and I kept on thinking why I hadn't done it before. Those 9 months were really special and have changed my life in various ways. My priorities, my lifestyle, and my overall outlook towards life have experienced a sea change. My son is 4 now and he's the joy of our lives, bringing smiles to our faces everyday.

With the baby growing inside you, and the hormonal changes along with it, there are lots of symptoms you might experience. Well, you can write a whole book on pregnancy but here I just want to touch upon some basic problems faced by pregnant women. This includes morning sickness, constipation, dizziness, fatigue, insomnia, indigestion, changes in the shape and size of breasts, backache, heartburn and so on. To deal with all these, proper nutrition and exercise are extremely important during pregnancy. For morning sickness, you should eat something first thing in the morning when you wake up, be it a banana or a biscuit. You need to listen to your body and understand its signals. Walking and regular exercise together with a good diet does help to deal with the rest of the symptoms.

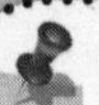

Stretch marks

Stretch marks are extremely common during and after pregnancy as the skin stretches a lot during this period. There are lots of products available in the market to deal with it, but one of the most effective solutions is to apply almond oil, twice

(*Cont.*)

a day, regularly. You should start this from the first trimester and not wait for the last minute. This will help in avoiding these marks on your body and will keep your skin as flawless as before. In some cases however it is hereditary and no matter how you take care you may still get stretch marks on your body. So here's wishing you good luck!

Pregnancy and becoming a mother was delightful but on the downside I had put on a lot of weight, almost 30 kilos. I was on bedrest for a few months after my delivery and funnily enough I put on a lot of weight after my baby was born as well. I was depressed and did not want to look at myself in the mirror. My body had changed and I missed slipping into my old clothes. I was desperate to lose weight and look and feel like before.

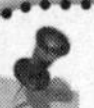

Having kids after 30

These days a lot of women are having kids in their thirties. There are several reasons for it but this is mainly because women in the cities are getting married late and are also ambitious about their careers now. However, when it comes to having a baby, age plays an important role and most doctors I spoke to tell me how it gets difficult to conceive after 35. Even if you do, there is a greater risk of abnormalities and extra care has to be taken at every stage.

New mums in their 30s also have a lot of stamina and resilience, qualities that come in handy for parenting young children. Everyone's different, of course, but you're likely to know yourself better than you did when you were in your 20s. You're also likely to be more flexible than you will be in your 40s.

It took me more than a year to get back into shape, but I was determined to get back into my old pair of jeans and I am happy to share that I managed to do that. You can too. Here are a few exercises you can do to lose the post pregnancy weight.

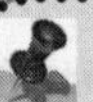

Workout for losing post pregnancy weight

A new mother should start slow and then progress; here are a few exercises you should start off with:

- Ashwinmudra (Pelvic contractions while inhaling and exhaling): This mudra involves making small contractions of the muscles at the vaginal wall. This helps strengthen weak pelvic muscles, which can cause bladder control issues, which are common in women postpartum.
- Walking: With your doctor's go ahead, short, slow walks can help prepare your body for more vigorous exercise, as well as get you fresh air. If you exercised before pregnancy, you may need about six weeks before you can return to what you were doing before.
- Yoga: Gentle yoga poses can be a great way to get your blood flowing while reducing stress. You may need to avoid some poses, but basic moves like Setubandhasana, Virabhadrasana (Warrior 1) and pelvic tilts, are a great place to start. You may also be able to find a postpartum yoga class at a local gym or health club.
- Breastfeeding is a very important factor in losing weight, you should ideally feed your baby for 6-8 months.

(*Cont.*)

Thereafter move on to the following workout:

Total time: 1 hour 15 minutes
Best time to do it: Morning on an empty stomach or evening after a gap of 4-5 hours after your meal

Warm up 5 minutes
Suryanamaskar 5 rounds (extremely slow to start with + 5 every week)
Tadasana 15 seconds each leg, 2 rounds each
Side bending Chakrasana 15 seconds each side, 2 rounds each
Veerbhadrasana 15 seconds, 2 rounds
Trikonasana 15 seconds, 2 rounds
Paschimottanasana 15 seconds, 2 rounds
Naukasana 15 seconds, 5 rounds
Setubandhasana 15 seconds, 2 rounds
Ushtarasana 15 seconds each side, 2 rounds
Suptvajrasana 15 seconds, 1 round
Pawanmuktasana 15 seconds each leg, 3 rounds each
Bhujangasana 10 seconds, 3 rounds
Dhanurasana 10 seconds, 3 rounds
Sarpasana 10 seconds, 3 rounds
Shavasana 2 minutes
Anulom Vilom 3 rounds
Om chanting 3 rounds

These tips may help you achieve and maintain a healthy weight:

- Make time for your meals, especially breakfast. Skipping meals can lower your energy levels and won't help you lose weight.
- Eat at least five portions of fruit and vegetables in a day.

(*Cont.*)

- Include plenty of fibre-rich foods such as vegetables, oats, lentils, and grains in your diet.
- Go easy on the special high-calorie foods given to women after birth, such as panjiri, ghee-laden dishes and fried dry fruit. Enjoy these tasty treats by balancing them with your meals. If you're eating a low-calorie meal such as khichdi, then you can go for a high-calorie til ka ladoo. But if you're eating aloo puri for lunch, you may want to save the panjiri for later.
- Watch your portions at mealtimes. Small meals eaten often can help prevent overeating.
- Drink plenty of low-calorie fluids like water, coconut water, and fresh fruit juices. Lots of calories can be hidden in packaged juices, full cream milk, and soft drinks.
- Breastfeed your baby. Experts say that exclusive breastfeeding makes it easier to regain your pre-pregnancy shape.
- Keep an eye on the number and type of snacks you have between meals. Opt for healthy and filling snacks like salads, fruit platters, or a glass of toned milk.

Position 8 of **Suryanamaskar, Parvatasana** and **Sarvangasana** are ideal postures during the postnatal recovery stage. They counteract the gravity effect on the internal organs during pregnancy. They also bring back these organs to their original positions. In the postnatal recovery stage, regular practice of Sarvangasana corrects enlargement of the ovary and the uterus.

Shavasana cures the sacroiliac joints which generally become rather tender and cause pain after delivery. These joints are required to be separated during the pelvic separation process during childbirth.

When we are in our mid-twenties going on to the mid-thirties, there is a lot going on in our lives. During this stage of their lives, women invariably juggle multiple roles and reset their priorities. For many of you, your careers would be taking shape while some of you would have graduated to the next level in your personal lives with marriage and kids. It is indeed a hectic time but also a critical period when you should not ignore your health. Inculcate good habits, make smart lifestyle choices, and learn to listen to your body. I know it's easy to get lost in the chaos of life but I hope this chapter will help you to make health a priority and understand its long term benefits.

BEFORE MENOPAUSE (35–45 YEARS)

This chapter is about the tricky mid-thirties and beyond. By now most of you would have made your choices of career, family and would have somewhat fixed habits. So if you have been exercising regularly and are conscious of your health you will find it easier to continue to stay on the right course. However if you have neither exercised nor played a sport ever in your life, you will need a lot of determination to make lifestyle changes. The good thing is that it's never too late to start and you can always acquire good habits.

Suman Mehta is 44, and a mother of two teenaged children. She was a successful jewellery designer in her twenties but when she became a mum she decided to be a homemaker and focus on her children. A totally devoted mum, her life would revolve around her 2 children. Somewhere along the line she stopped caring about her health and her body, always putting family first. As a result she put on weight and today she looks probably 55 instead of her real age. This is not an isolated example and I'm sure there are many more Sumans around us. I have written this chapter especially for such selfless mums and would like them to start caring for themselves. You owe it to yourself. Remember, you can make others happy only if you feel joyful inside.

Being a mum

Motherhood is a very special feeling. Out of all the roles a woman plays, being a mother is probably the one that most women cherish the most. It is also a defining moment and challenging too as it involves a different approach and acquiring new skills. A mother not just nurtures the child but also teaches her baby values that shape the intellect and personality. You have to understand not just yourself and your body but also the needs of your child.

A lot of women get married late unlike earlier days when most girls were married off by the time they turned 25. Women today want to wait for the right partner, make their career and take the plunge into matrimony when they feel ready. Getting married in the thirties or mid-thirties is very common now and consequently a lot of women plan to have babies around their mid-thirties or even later. Advancing age and modern lifestyle has given a spurt to several fertility issues. Who would believe it would be difficult to have babies in a country like India? But times have changed and so have issues around women's health. Stress is, as they say, one of the best contraceptives. Daily worries, tension and work or home pressure is also responsible for infertility besides medical causes. In the box I have outlined a basic workout for infertility related to stress.

Workout for tackling infertility

If the cause is medical, please consult a doctor.
If the cause is stress, you could do the following workout.

Total time: 1 hour excluding the walking time
Best time to do it: Morning on an empty stomach or evening after a gap of 4-5 hours after your meal

30 minute happy walking (think about everything that makes you happy)
Warm up for 5 minutes
Suryanamaskar with breath concentration, 1 round
Deep breathing: Focus on deep inhalation or exhalation, 5 times
Vrikshasana hold for 10 seconds, 2 rounds
Natrajasana hold for 10 seconds, 2 rounds
Garudasana hold for 10 seconds, 2 rounds

Sitting asanas
Parvatasana hold for 10 seconds, 2 rounds
Yogmudra hold for 10 seconds, 2 rounds
Matsyasana hold for 10 seconds, 2 rounds

Lying down (supine)
Pavanmuktasana hold for 10 seconds, 2 rounds
Sarvangasana hold for 15 seconds, 1 round
Counterpose, Setubandhasana, 1 round

Lying down (prone)
Dhanurasana hold for 10 seconds, 2 rounds
Makarasana relaxation for 2 minutes
Bhramari Pranayam, 5 times
Om or any other chanting, 5 times

Forties is the new Thirties

Ever since I became a mother, my life has changed completely. My world now revolves around my little bundle of joy. I recently turned forty and I must tell you, the journey so far has been fantastic. Through ups and downs, life has changed dramatically. There have been fewer sad moments and a lot of happy ones. Every morning when I wake up, I feel it is a new beginning, a new day to explore and learn more. Motherhood becomes central to the life of most 35-45 year old women. Lifestyles, location and language may differ, but I am sure most of you who is in this age group has a similar story to tell.

I often say that Forties is the new Thirties especially when we are surrounded by gorgeous mums like Malaika Arora Khan, Maria Goretti and Farah Khan. I often tell fellow mums that motherhood is not the end of your life and not an excuse to lose control of your body. I see a lot of women around me who stop caring about themselves and their bodies once they have children. They become overweight, look older than their age and are often tired all the time. Wake up! You need to get back to being healthy and looking good. You owe it to yourself. The truth is that we all can do it. It might take more effort than it took you when you were sixteen but you can still fit into your old pair of jeans and look attractive. If you are slightly overweight, you could follow the below workout to get to your ideal weight. You could lose the extra weight in three months if you follow the regimen regularly and watch your diet at the same time.

Workout to lose less than 8 kilos

Total time: 1 hour excluding the walking time
Best time to do it: Morning on an empty stomach or evening after a gap of 4-5 hours after your meal

1. **Morning walk** 30 to 45 minutes (Everyday)
2. Jalneti, thrice a month
3 Shankhprakchalana, twice a month
4. Kapalabhati, 200 to 300 times everyday
5. **Workout** (Thrice a week, alternate days)
a. Suryanamaskar, 25 rounds
b. 25 sit-ups, 2 rounds
c. 25 sidekicks, with each leg, 2 rounds
d. 50 upper crunches, 2 rounds
e. 25 leg raises, 4 rounds
f. Naukasana, 15 seconds, 2 rounds
g. Dhanurasana, 15 seconds, 2 rounds
h. Shavasana, 5 minutes

6. **Pranayam**
a. Anulom Vilom, 5 to 10 rounds
b. Ujjyai, 5 to 10 rounds

The below workout is for women who are more than 8 kilos overweight and want to get back into shape. Depending on how many kilos you need to lose, you will have to continue the workout for as many months. Don't lose hope; make a start and you will get there eventually. You could take a picture of yourself every month to inspire yourself in this journey for good health. Believe me it works!

Workout to lose more than 8 kilos

Total time: 1 hour excluding the walking time

Best time to do it: Morning on an empty stomach or evening after a gap of 4-5 hours after your meal

Tip: Beginners who have never exercised should not attempt full workouts and follow the advice of an expert

1. **Morning walk**

5 minutes, normal walk
2 minutes, normal running
(8 to 10 rounds)

2. Vaman kriya, twice a week
3. Shankhprakshalana, every week for two months
4. Kapalabhati kriya, 300 to 500 times everyday
5. **Workouts (Four days in a week)**

a. 5 sit-ups with front kicks, 5 rounds
b. 25 lunges with each leg, 2 rounds
c. 50 sidekicks against the wall with each leg, 2 rounds
d. 25 push-ups on your knees, 2 rounds
e. Santolanasana, 15 seconds, 2 rounds
f. 25 upper crunches+ 25 leg raises, 4 rounds
g. Triyak Naukasana on each side, 15 seconds, 2 rounds
h. Naukasana, 15 seconds, 2 rounds
i. Naukasana in prone position, 15 seconds, 2 rounds
j. Shavasana, 5 minutes

6. **Pranayam**

a. Anulom Vilom, 5 rounds
b. Bhramari, 10 rounds
c. Om chanting, 5 rounds

Walking the tightrope

Balancing motherhood, career and family can seem an impossibly difficult job, but it isn't really so. A lot of women do it and do it well. Women are great at multitasking and wearing different hats. It comes naturally to us, doesn't it? Cooking dinner, watching TV, while making sure the child is doing the homework all at the same time. Caring for children is is probably more time consuming and draining if they are young. How they keep us on our toes constantly. My 4-year-old son is partly responsible for keeping me fit running as I am around him most of the time, playing games with him, taking him out for walks, ferrying him from school and so on.

It is easy to get lost in the midst of all this activity and find that you have no time for yourself. The most important thing in these cases is to get organized. Make sure that you have everything in place so that you do not waste time looking for them. Assign particular places for toys, books, clothes, and so on. Maintain a to-do list or calendar and mark all important dates. Keep essential items like keys, mobile phone, office documents in an assigned place. If your child is in junior school, keep the uniform ironed, bag packed, and shoes ready the night before. Try easy to make recipes for the tiffin.

Teach your child to be independent and organized too, keeping things in place. Teach these important lessons early on. If your work hours are too demanding, spend time with your child on weekends. Go out for some fun activity that can be done together. Why not try painting, singing, dancing, or just doing chores like cleaning together? In the midst of running around if you feel you get a headache quite often or have migraine you could try this workout.

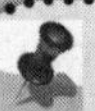

Workout for migraine

Total time: The time and number of rounds will vary as per the severity of your problem, and as recommended by the expert

Best time to do it: Morning on an empty stomach or evening after a gap of 4-5 hours after your meal

1. Padahastasana
2. Vipreetkarni
3. Sarwangasana
4. Shirshasana

Pranayama

1. Suryabhedan
2. Bhastirika
3. Bhramari

Kriya

1. Kunjal
2. Jalneti
3. Trataka
4. Kapalabhati

Bandha

1. Mulabandh

Being the mother of a teenager can be extremely challenging. Sporadic moods and emotional outrages can be really difficult to handle. You need to be patient with your kid. It is extremely important to open up to your child and talk to him. Be a friend rather than a strict disciplinarian. Communication is very important. We all have gone through this phase. Give wings to your children's imagination and let them grow.

One of the things that I recommend a lot of women in this age group is to find an hour only for themselves first thing in the morning before you get drowned in the chaos of the day. This is extremely useful to gather your thoughts, prepare for the day ahead, listen to your body and focus on your priorities. If you could use this time to exercise, it is even better. This one hour can change your life and if you do it regularly you will realize how it will make a difference in everything that you do. Every morning when I wake up, I think about the day ahead; the important things on my to-do list, then go out for a quick walk or do my workout. During this time when my home is relatively quiet I feel I can think about myself, how I'm feeling in my body and my mind. I want to stay fit and happy to bring joy to my home and this one hour helps me in achieving it.

Early signs of ageing

Most women notice the first signs of ageing around the mid-thirties. Greying hair, fine lines around the eyes, dark circles, wrinkles, hair fall, loose or dull skin, change in posture, and lack of vigour are commonly faced by most 35–45-year-olds. You are slowly moving towards menopause and hence hormonal changes can lead to psychological as well as physical changes in your body. You need to understand that these changes are quite natural and there's nothing to feel scared about. One of the common issues faced by women due to hormonal imbalance is thyroid. Do you feel tired all the time, feel bloated and perhaps have gained weight very quickly over the past few months? If the answer is yes, you should consult a doctor. You could also do the workout below which can help you in dealing with thyroid.

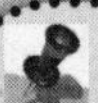

Workout for thyroid

Total time: The time and number of rounds will vary as per the severity of your problem, and as recommended by the expert
Best time to do it: Morning on an empty stomach or evening after a gap of 4-5 hours after your meal

1. Matsyasana
2. Brahammudra
3. Vipreetkarni
4. Sarwangasana
5. Poorna Halasana
6. Chakrasana

Pranayama
1. Ujjayi
2. Bhramari
3 Anulom Vilom

Bandha
1. Jalandhara Bandha

Grey hair

Remember your first grey hair? That day when you woke up, looked at yourself in the mirror and suddenly found a grey speck staring back at you? I am sure you do. Do you know why our hair greys? As we age, the production of melanin in our hair follicles slows down. Now you'll ask, what's melanin? Melanin is a pigment that gives colour to your hair. You cannot stop your hair from greying since it is triggered genetically but you can surely maintain the health of your hair. Here are some home remedies to stop our hair from greying.

- Eat protein-rich foods such as whole grains, chicken, soy, eggs, and cereals.
- Have an amla everyday.
- Foods rich in iron like green leafy veggies, bananas, tomatoes, and yogurt can also help.
- Iodized table salt is important for the production of melanin.
- Do not stress yourself.
- Try out yoga.

Dark circles

I often say dark circles are a beauty killer. You might be slim and feel energetic but if you have these shadows around your eyes you will look tired. Dark circles can add years to your face and make you look older even faster than wrinkles or grey hair. Why do we get dark circles? Lack of proper sleep, insomnia, lethargy, allergy, and diet imbalance primarily induce dark pigmentation around our eyes. Are there ways to prevent these annoying shadows under the eyes? Here are a few things you can try.

- Refrigerate used teabags and place them on your eyes for 5 minutes as often as possible. You can also use cucumber slices or a chilled muslin cloth for this.
- Proper sleep for around 6-8 hours is essential. Sleep in a comfortable, properly ventilated, dark room. Do not have coffee, alcohol, or tea before going to bed.
- Drink at least eight glasses of water everyday.
- Neti Kriya can also help you relieve dark circles.

Wrinkles

As your skin ages, it becomes thinner and drier and loses much of its elasticity. Over time skin produces less oil and the body's natural moisture is reduced causing wrinkles. Wrinkles and lines first appear near the eyes and mouth, and gradually move up to the forehead, throat, and neck areas. Proper and regular moisturizing can help reduce wrinkles. Here are a few home remedies that can be tried.

- Fish is an excellent source of nutrients that can nourish the skin. If you are vegetarian try the omega supplements as recommended by your doctor.
- Use a good facial lotion that contains mineral oils. A gentle water-based moisturizer can actually help reduce wrinkles.
- Foods that contain soy can also be helpful. You can try a variety of soy-based foods like milk, tofu, meat products, cereals, and breads.
- Beat 2 egg whites and apply it on your face as a mask. Let it dry for 30 minutes and then rinse your face with cold water.
- Multani mitti or kaolin clay powder mixed with water can also be applied as a face pack.
- Honey mixed with two teaspoons of full cream milk can smoothen your skin and help fade fine lines.

35-45 is an important stage in every woman's life and also the time when things can go wrong. You may start ignoring yourself physically and mentally, face health issues and lose the lust for life. On the other hand, you can also use this stage to stay fit (and win compliments ☺), set your priorities right and cultivate good habits or hobbies. Who doesn't want to hear that they look younger? It's every woman's dream and wish to look and feel desirable especially during this tricky stage. So let's not slip and fall but use yoga as a friend to guide us on our journey to health and happiness.

AFTERGLOW
(BEYOND 45 YEARS)

We can't deny that as time passes our bodies too undergo change. Let's face it. There are things in our control and then there are some which we can't duck. Heredity, injuries, and genetic conditions can affect anyone and especially women after 45 as the body ages and loses the resistance of a 16-year-old. If your grandparents or parents had diabetes, you also may be at a risk. Nonetheless, you can safeguard your health by controlling your decisions and lifestyle choices. All of us are unique and the natural process of ageing affects each one of us in different ways. To understand age related problems, you must try and listen to your body. Try and understand its signals—how it functions, what are the needs of your body. You must also follow a fitness or health routine that befits your mental and physical requirements. Habits and choices are purely yours. All you need to do is integrate healthy habits and beneficial choices in your lifestyle.

When health is priceless

We all grow older and whether we like it or not it is a fact of life. The right attitude is to embrace it and try to enjoy it. Once you cross the age of 45, a number of diseases like blood pressure, arthritis, fibroids, obesity, and diabetes crop up. Most women beyond 45 have some or the other health concern and I feel it is important to manage our fitness carefully than ever before. For me there is nobody who epitomizes this better than Sridevi. She is beautiful, fit, strong, and graceful. Even more now than ever before. She does yoga regularly, paints, spends time with family and loves trying out new things. Life is about living in the moment and enjoying every bit of it.

By this time, most of you would have settled down, enjoyed motherhood, and now be treading towards the dreaded path of menopause. Some of you would have gone through menopause already. In this stage of our life, the body undergoes transformation—your hormones no longer function the way they did during the childbearing years. Many women undergo symptoms like hot flashes, stress, lack of libido, depression, night sweats, urinary infection, insomnia, anxiety, vaginal itching, mood swings, weight gain, irritability, and hopelessness. As ageing progresses your body's resistance to health conditions and immunity deteriorates. You become susceptible to diseases and health problems crop up. Sleeping disorders and weak eyesight are also common once you cross 50.

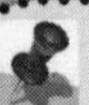

Workout for joint pain

Total time: The time and number of rounds will vary as per the severity of your problem, and as recommended by the expert
Best time to do it: Morning on an empty stomach or evening after a gap of 4-5 hours after your meal

1. Parvatasana
2. Utkatasana

(*Cont.*)

3. Garudasana
4. Goumukhasana
5. Matsyendrasana
6. Bhadrasana
7. Vajrasana
8. Padmasana

Pranayam

1. Anulom Vilom
2. Bhramari

Menopause

How we all dread this word! Before we move further, let us try and understand what menopause actually means. Why is there so much fear and misconception about menopause? How can we deal with it well? Remember, there is no running away from it. The term menopause is derived from the words 'men' which means month and 'pausis' which means termination. Caused by the natural degeneration of reproductive hormones in the body, menopause is a transition which marks the end of a woman's fertility and her menstrual cycles. Surgical removal of the uterus and ovaries can also cause menopause. Most women experience it either in their late 40s or their early 50s.

For a very long time, women believed that menopause is the end of life or at least the end of their sex life. Do not panic as it is only the end of your reproductive life. Meena Gupta, 58 is a housewife and has been enjoying an even better sex life after menopause. She feels she has more time with her husband now that her kids are married and settled. They take regular holidays, communicate better and still feel attracted to each other. Yes, its true that there may be issues like vaginal dryness and so on but there are solutions for these. So let's not feel sad thinking about menopause and look at it as another milestone in our life.

Before its onset or during perimenopause, most women experience some or a few of these symptoms.

- Hot Flashes

It is the most common symptom associated with menopause experienced by almost 75 percent women. It lasts from 30 seconds to a few minutes. Hot flashes increase the body temperature causing excessive perspiration, agitation, lightheadedness, nausea, heart palpitations, and breathlessness. There is a sudden flushing of the face as the area around the head and neck reddens.

- Night Sweats

These are hot flashes that occur while sleeping especially at night time. Hormonal fluctuations are the main cause for it. Night sweats can interrupt sleep and can hence be extremely annoying. You can control night sweats by taking a cool shower before going to bed, eating a balanced diet, drinking lots of water, avoiding alcohol and smoking, and sleeping in a cool room.

- Vaginal Dryness

It is a common problem faced by more than 80 percent women during perimenopause. Decreased lubrication causes this problem. Since lubrication and moisture helps keep harmful bacteria at bay, many women may face yeast infection, vaginal itching, painful intercourse, and urinary tract infection due to vaginal dryness. Some women may experience loss of libido which is aggravated due to the lack of adequate vaginal moisture. Lack of libido can also result in the thinning of vaginal walls causing painful intercourse. But the good news is that yoga can help you rejuvenate your sexual life.

- Irregular Periods

As we move towards menopause, hormonal fluctuations increase, causing irregular periods. Some women may also skip their periods or not have them at all. If your period stops and does not occur for over a year, you have reached the state of menopause.

Since menopause is inevitable and something I want all women to embrace rather than dread, let's look at a few exercises that can help us during this phase.

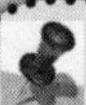

Workout for menopause

Total time: 1 hour

Best time to do it: Morning on an empty stomach or evening after a gap of 4-5 hours after your meal

Tip: Kriyas and bandhas should be practiced under the guidance of an expert

1. Jalneti Kriya
2. Kapalabhati Kriya, 100 times, 2 rounds with 30 seconds interval
3. Trataka Kriya, till your eyes blink, 2 rounds

(*Cont.*)

4. Uddiyaan Bandha, hold for 15 seconds, 2 rounds
5. Postures- All postures to be held for 15 seconds, 2 rounds each

Standing asanas

a. Tadasana
b. Parvatasana
c. Trikonasana
d. Natrajasana

Sitting asanas

a. Paschimottanasana
b. Vakrasana
c. Supta Vajrasana
d. Bhadrasana

Supine position

a. Vipreetkarni
b. Sarvangasana
c. Poorna Halasana
d. Setubandhasana

Prone position

a. Dhanurasana
b. Shalabhasana
c. Bhujangasana
d. Makarasana

6. **Pranayam**

a. Anulom Vilom, 5 rounds
b. Ujjyai, 10 rounds
c. Bhramari, 10 rounds
d. Om chanting, 10 rounds

7. **Relaxation**

a. Shavasana, 5 minutes

Fibroids

Fibroids are generally non-cancerous, fibrous tumors that occur in the uterus. They are usually harmless but can nonetheless cause abnormal bleeding, constipation, urinary disorders, abdominal bloating, lower back pain, and pelvic pain. I recommend that women in their 40s visit their gynaecologist at least once a year for a check up. Fibroids can lead to discomfort and soreness and hence aggravate problems related to perimenopause. But the good news is that its occurrence shrinks after menopause.

Consuming too much alcohol, red meat, and soy products enhances the chances of developing fibroids. Include a lot of green, leafy vegetables in your diet. Drinking a glass of milk everyday can also help reduce the risk. You must have at least 8 glasses of water and practice Pranayam every day.

Feeling 16

There are a lot of ways that can help you look and feel young. The most important is positive attitude. If your attitude towards life is right and you are positive, you can achieve anything. Everything depends on how you handle difficulties. Old age is actually beautiful. It is the time when you can sit back and relax and see your worries melt away. What could be better than seeing your efforts being paid off? You can spoil the peace of your mind by cribbing, thinking about what you don't have and lamenting endlessly. This is the time to feel good by doing things you like. You might be ailing and tired of the constant drill of life and its pressures but you should learn to greet whatever comes your way with a smile. With age, youth fades and you cannot revitalize it but you can always remain young at heart. Here are a few things you can do to look and feel younger:

- Take good care of yourself. Never depend upon anyone else for it. Do it yourself.
- Wear clothes that suit you and look good on you.
- If exercising is not your cup of tea, try walking. Go out for a nature walk. It'll help you detoxify and will make you feel fresh. Believe me, brisk walking is one of the best exercises and suitable for all ages.
- Practice yoga every morning. Try pranayam and other simple breathing exercises to feel invigorated and energized.
- Since laughter is the best medicine you can join a laughter club. Laughing out aloud not only enlivens your spirit but also makes you feel super energized. Or simply watch your favourite comedy soap.
- Pursue a hobby. Join a club where like-minded people can meet and discuss things that define your lives and passions. You and your friends can open up your own club and meet regularly. Books, nature, food, sketching, photography, singing, fitness, art, travel, social service—anything can be your inspiration.
- Interact with people. Talk to your children. Enjoy the company of old friends and make new ones. Conversation is the key to happiness.
- Old age is also the best time for your spiritual awakening. Meditation can help you channelize your energy and direct it towards positivity.
- Aroma therapy can be extremely beneficial to feel energized.
- Avoid wear heavy makeup. It can make you look older.
- Never underestimate yourself. Be natural and feel confident.

- Drink at least 8 glasses of water everyday.
- With age comes compassion and understanding. Forgive and forget is the key to contentment. Let go of people who do not care for you and things you cannot change.
- Enjoy the feeling of being a grandmother. Spend quality time with your grandchildren. Go out with them.
- Diet is very important. Do not eat oily and spicy food. Keep a tab on your health. Avoid sweets. Have at least one green leafy vegetable and one fruit a day. Dinner should always be light.
- Avoid consuming alcohol. Do not drink more than two cups of tea or coffee in a day.
- Your muscles need to be relaxed. Massage your body at least once in every two weeks. This is a great method of increasing blood circulation. You can also visit a nearby spa to unwind and relax.

Home remedies for wrinkles and ageing skin

There are plenty of home remedies that you might have heard about or even tried. Here are a few that I swear by and would recommend:

1. For glow and removing dark circles: Mix equal measure of yogurt, honey, vitamin E oil and lemon juice. Apply it on your face and leave it on for 15 minutes, then wash it off.
2. For wrinkles: Two of the best tricks to delay wrinkles is washing your face daily with water mixed with rosewater and then applying sandalwood paste made with rubbing the stick on a stone base at home.
3. For firmness: Use a papaya pack made with its pulp and apply it on your face. Leave it on for 15 minutes before washing it off. It works wonders.

Ageing with grace

Stories may differ but most women in their 60s and 70s feel the pangs of solitude and loneliness. They feel unhappy and crave for sentiments that can fill their emotional void. But why is it so? Old age is inevitable and will eventually embrace each one of us. Then why don't we welcome it gracefully? Living with contentment is much better than living with regrets. With age comes understanding and wisdom. Do not let unhappiness and dissatisfaction govern your life. Try to find pleasure in little things. Fit in pieces of happiness into the larger canvas of your life and everything around you will turn beautiful. For a sound body and mind, maintaining good health and fitness is vital. Preserving one's beauty and grace is upto you. I meet a lot of celebrity grannies who look stunning. Who doesn't want to look as elegant as a Waheeda Rahman or a Helen? We all look up to these women and often wonder what keeps them ticking. They not only look charming and elegant but are also fit. Even in old age they retain a charismatic youthfulness. If they can do it, so can you. Want to know their secret? I'll tell you how.

Community living

As I said, it is never too late to try new things. Why let age come in the way of pursuing your hobbies and interests? Interests can help you attain afterglow, the beauty of ageing. Here's a list of some activities that you can start and some awesome hobbies you can try.

- Movie club: Are you a big fan of Hitchcock or Woody Allen? Do you love Hindi movies? If yes, this hobby will surely interest you. Why not start a movie club? Form a group of

(*Cont.*)

like-minded friends and watch your favourite movies every weekend. You can also select movies by genre or actors. In one session you can watch thrillers and then switch to Audrey Hepburn's movies in the next session.

- Cooking and baking: I am sure most of you love cooking. So why not pursue this hobby to try out new things? Why not make delicious cupcakes, lasagna, cheesecake, pasta, chocolate, or awesome dips? You can also watch videos on YouTube and learn exotic recipes from around the world. Now that sounds interesting, doesn't it? A scrumptious treat for your family, friends, and yourself. Also, a great way to impress people. What say?
- Fitness on the go: Who doesn't want to look good and feel fit? We all want to have fab bodies like Kareena Kapoor and Sridevi. So why not transform this fitness activity into a hobby and do it with friends? Why not practice yoga everyday? Wouldn't it be wonderful if your interest and fitness mantra become the same? Try it and see it work for yourself.
- Book club and reading: Book club can be an awesome way to rewind and relax for all the book lovers. You can either join public libraries if you love reading or start your own book club with a group of friends with similar interests. You can have interactive sessions, book reviews, and discussions about genres and authors.
- Gardening: Who doesn't love nature? What could be better than bringing home nature's bounty? Gardening can be an extremely interesting way to interact and connect to the environment. Potting plants, planting seeds, growing flowers, and pruning can be a wonderful way to relax your senses.
- DIY Projects: Do-it-yourself projects are simply amazing. You can browse the internet and find hordes of such projects. So be it pottery or sculpting, art and craft or photo editing, you can now do exciting new things! You have the time for it so use it creatively.

Life comes full circle

Husband, children, and family form the locus of every woman's life. After 45, these relationships seem all the more fragile and need to be handled with love and care. As you age, accepting life and its problems becomes all the more difficult. Children grow up and settle down, reproductive age ends, physical needs take a backseat, and social and psychological needs become vital. Here are a few things that can help you build good relationships and enjoy your old age.

- Spending time with family members not only enhances healthier relationships but can also strengthen interpersonal bonds. Acceptance and trust is equally vital.
- Follow a balanced diet that makes you feel healthy as well as happy. Include lots of fruits and veggies.
- Embrace ageing gracefully. Keeping alive the spark of romance is equally important. Avocados, basil, bananas, and almonds can help increase libido.
- Adore your changing body. Your appearance might change after menopause but accepting yourself the way you are is very important. If you do not accept yourself, how would others accept you? Never ever underestimate yourself.
- Discuss your problems with your husband and try and understand his needs.
- Exercise daily. Go out for morning or evening walk with your hubby or children. Practice yoga regularly.
- Provide support and guidance to your children. Stand by them when they face problems.
- Kickstart your morning with a glass of lukewarm water and have at least 8 glasses of water every day.

- Try out things you never imagined you'd do. Take the opportunity to experiment and learn new things. Try taking road trips, baking, knitting, painting, blogging, and so on. Just explore unexplored horizons.
- Celebrate the beauty of life. Ageing should not hamper your spirits. Do not let your life take a back seat.
- Involve yourself in family problems but also respect each other's personal space.
- Prioritize your work and home life. Spend ample time with people close to you. Meet your friends as much as you can.
- Have a positive attitude towards life. Accept challenges and never let any thing hamper your thought process.
- Lack of communication is the root cause of all problems. You must try and interact as much as you can. Honest discussions are good for bonding. Having lunch or dinner together with the family can also be a good option.
- Planning your retirement and accordingly setting up family goals can also help in the smooth functioning of the household.

When I was writing this chapter my thoughts would invariably go back to my mother who I feel is one of the most graceful women I know. The energy and enthusiasm she has reflects in her appearance and gives her an inner glow. How has she done it? What makes her look and feel good even in her sixties? Regular exercise, spiritual growth, and accepting the way we are are the most important factors according to her. I'm sure it will be different things for different women but we all can find our magic potion, the secret formula that works for us. Surprise yourself, get out of that couch and start walking on the road to becoming a Body Goddess. Let's join hands, support each other, and do it together.

ACKNOWLEDGEMENTS

Before I can even collect my thoughts, I would like to thank the almighty, the supreme power, for making me the medium to reach out to the world in my own little way through this book as well as my first book. I would like to express my gratitude to Sridevi Kapoor for her unstinting support, patiently reading drafts of the book, offering suggestions, and agreeing to write the foreword to the book. This book would have been incomplete without you. A big thank you to you!

I am deeply indebted to the readers of my debut book *From XL to XS*; followers on the Cosmic Fusion website and the Facebook page for writing to me and sharing your thoughts. Your comments and questions helped me improve the content of this book in a big way.

My celebrity clients who took out their valuable time to share their thoughts, tips and experiences and shoot pictures for the book. You have always been there for me.

My students for bearing with my irregular presence and their wholehearted support throughout the writing of this book.

I would like to thank Zoa Morani who generously volunteered to shoot for the yoga pictures in the book. Thank you for your love and support.

My friend and HR Manager Hemali Punjabi, my personal manager Jacqueline D'Almeida and all the teachers and staff at Cosmic Fusion for their whole hearted support by running the show when I needed the much needed time away to write this book.

My family who have always been a great support for everything in my life and stood by me in all my ventures.

My heartfelt gratitude goes to my parents for bringing me up and teaching me valuable life lessons. I have no words to thank you enough for all the love, relentless support you have offered in every venture in my life.

Milee Ashwarya, my editor, for taking the time to edit and lay this book out; for providing me with the inspiration to write my debut book and now *Body Goddess*. I appreciate you more than you'll ever know. Anukriti Sharma, Gurveen Chadha and Radhika Marwah for proofreading and improving the text with their inputs.

I would like to thank my husband Manish Tiwari for standing beside me through thick and thin, supporting my career and helping me in writing this book. He has been my inspiration and motivation for continuing to improve my knowledge and move ahead in my career. You are my rock, and I dedicate this book to you and our son Sayaan Tiwari. Thank you my little angel for always making me smile and for understanding on those weekend mornings when I was writing this book instead of playing games. I hope that one day you can read this book and understand why I spent so much time in front of my computer. Thank you my son for making me a mother and completing my life.

A NOTE ON THE AUTHOR

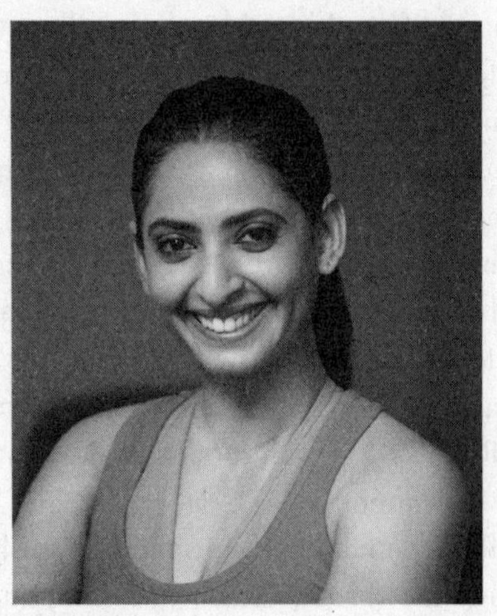

Payal Gidwani Tiwari is one of the most famous fitness and yoga experts of Bollywood. Her clients include Sridevi and Boney Kapoor, Kareena Kapoor, Sanjay and Karisma Kapoor, Rani Mukherji, Saif Ali Khan, Farhan Akhtar, Neelam Kothari, Susanne Roshan, Shaheen Abbas, Farah Khan, Vaibhavi Merchant, Shailendra Singh, Raju Manwani, Roopa Vohra, Divya Kohli, Rashmi Nigam, Shaana Dia, Jacqueline Fernandez, Malaika Arora Khan, Tusshar Kapoor, Ekta Kapoor, Amrita Arora Ladak, Laila Khan, Tulip Joshi, Maria Goretti, Zoa

Morani, Priya Dutt, Poorna Patel, Sonakshi Sinha, Dr Vijay Mallya, and Siddhart Malhotra.

She also conducts yoga workshops for corporates, and runs her own wellness brand called Cosmic Fusion (www.cosmicfusion.in), which emphasizes daily fitness and a holistic lifestyle. Payal was on the panel of judges for 'The Femina Miss India 2013' pageant. She judged the sub-contest and crowned Femina Miss India Body Beautiful 2013.

She is the author of the bestselling book *From XL to XS* which has sold more than 75,000 copies across the country.

ABOUT COSMIC FUSION

The studio Cosmic Fusion opened for classes in Jan 2010 and has become become one of Mumbai's most respected yoga studios. With a maximum in-studio class capacity of 25 students, Cosmic Fusion is a 'boutique' wellness brand at the forefront of yoga and wellness disciplines through conducting interactive sessions that enhance an individual's mind, body and soul.

Payal and Manish along with their team hold regular ongoing sessions at Cosmic Fusion which is a very eclectic place for imparting wellness disciplines. They have a trained team of enthusiastic individuals who make sure that every student in every session goes back with a much more open-minded outlook towards their individual lifestyles.

Payal is an individual who has always strived for reaching higher grounds. Having been qualified as an Interior Designer and worked on numerous assignments for a number of years; she finally had a spiritual calling and this made her turn to the holistic discipline of yoga. Payal soon started learning the ropes of one of the highest forms of spiritual discipline. Soon she was initiated as one of the foremost yoga masters in Mumbai and it was around this time that the very famous Bollywood actress Kareena Kapoor wanted to undergo a radical change in her personal lifestyle. Since then she has gone on to initiate Saif Ali Khan, Rani Mukherji amongst many others too.

Manish is a visionary and a yoga master. Having been spiritually inclined from early on, he left home for greener pastures to find his true self. This seeking within led him to the Kevalyadham Institute (one of the world's best Yoga research institutes); where he spent a complete year learning the craft of yoga and developing himself as an holistic individual.

He then came to Mumbai in 2002 and since then he has been at the forefront of spreading this wellness lifestyle of yoga to individuals, corporate and Bollywood celebs like Sridevi, Katrina Kaif amongst many others.

Address: 403, Saffier Building, 4th Floor, Santacruz (West) Linking Road Mumbai- 400054.

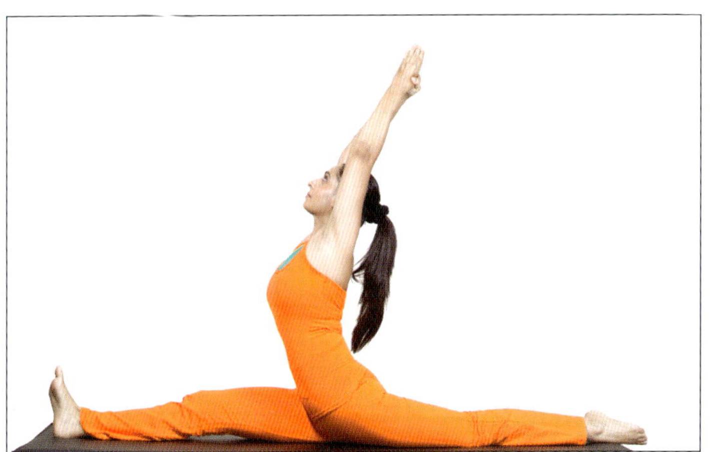

Hanuman Asana

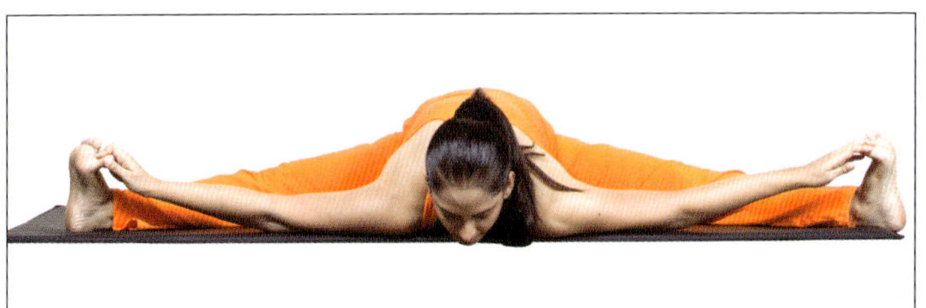

Ugrasana

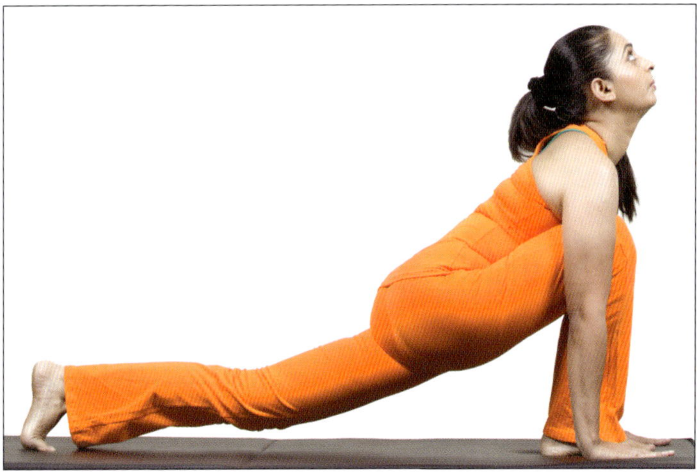

Ashwa Sanchalan Asana

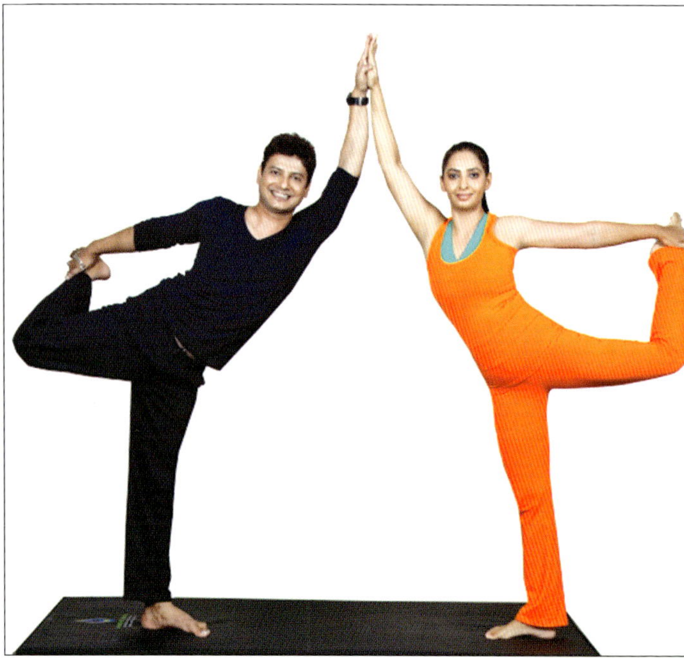

Couple Natrajasana

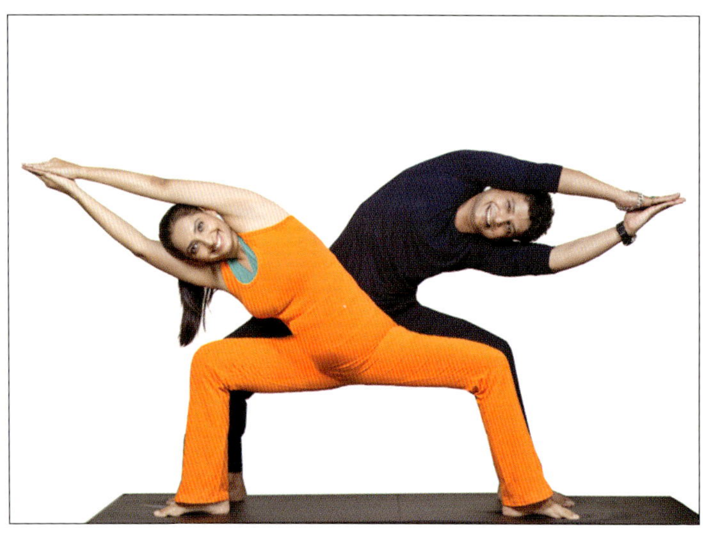

Couple Side Bending Chakrasana

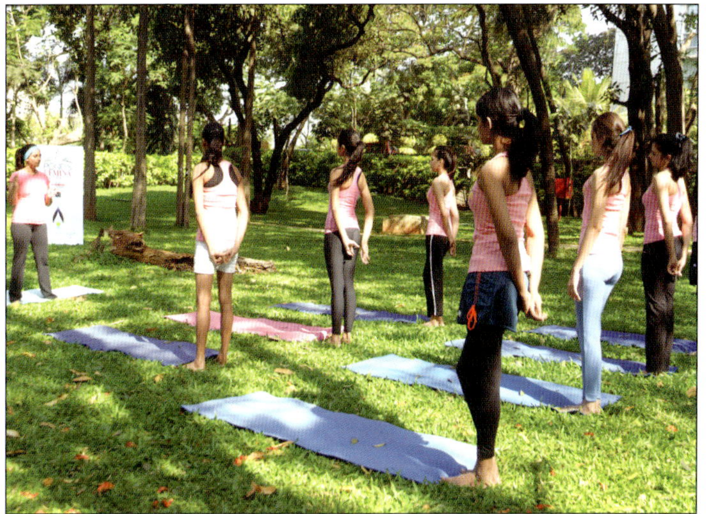

Teaching the Femina Miss India 2013 contestants

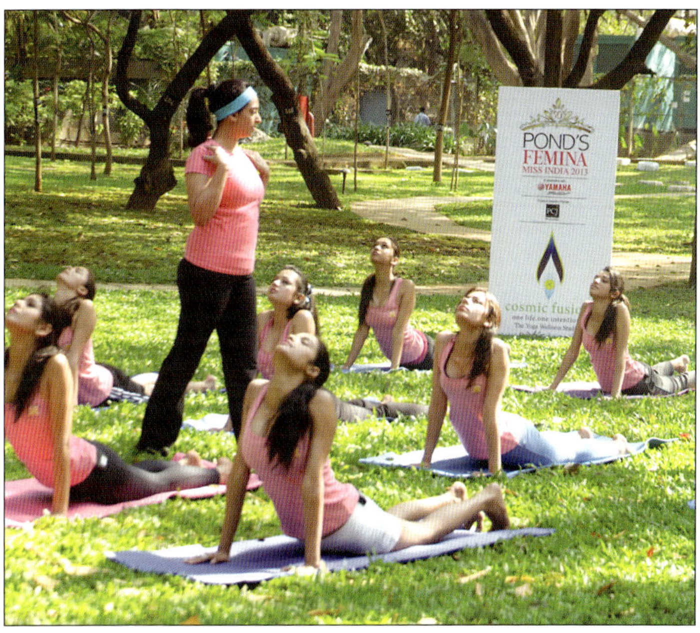

Teaching the Femina Miss India 2013 contestants Sarpasana

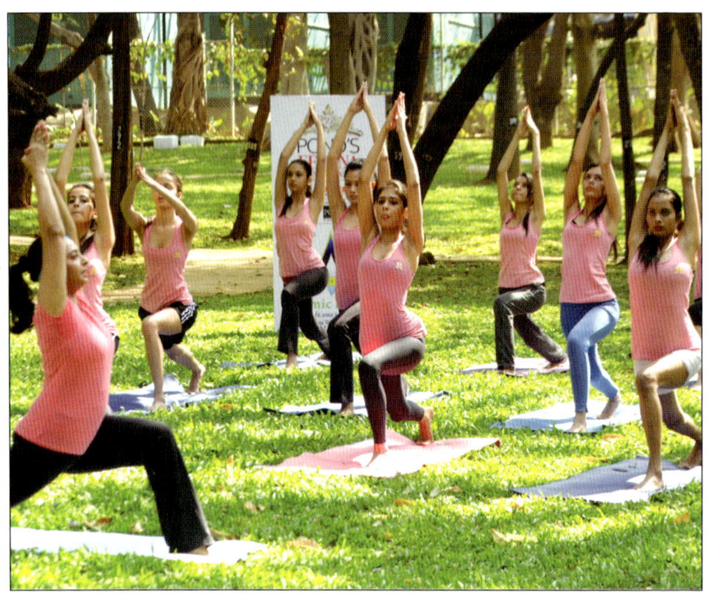

Teaching the Femina Miss India 2013 contestants Virasana

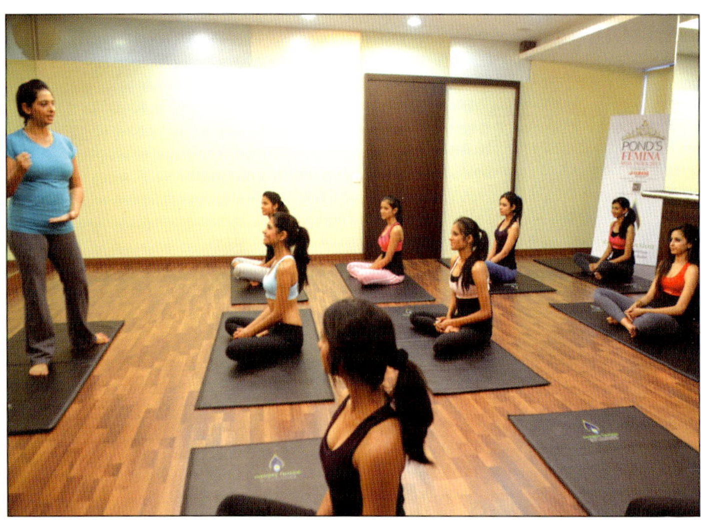

Teaching the Femina Miss India 2013 contestants at Cosmic Fusion, the Yoga Wellness Studio

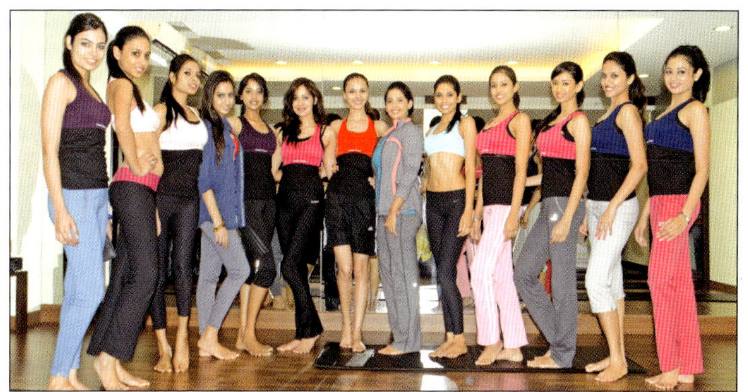

Teaching the Femina Miss India 2013 contestants at Cosmic Fusion, the Yoga Wellness Studio

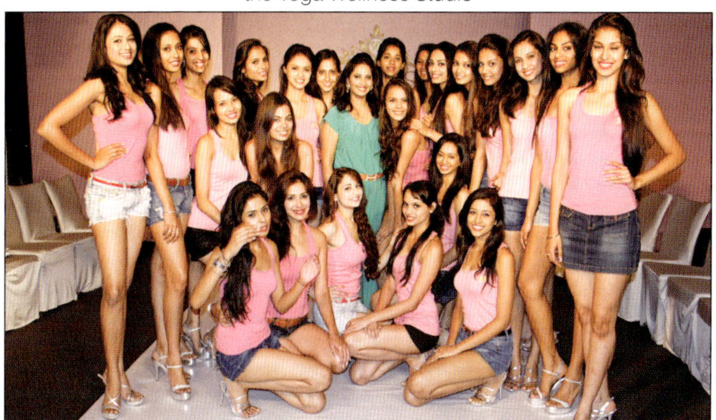

Judging Femina Miss Body Beautiful 2013

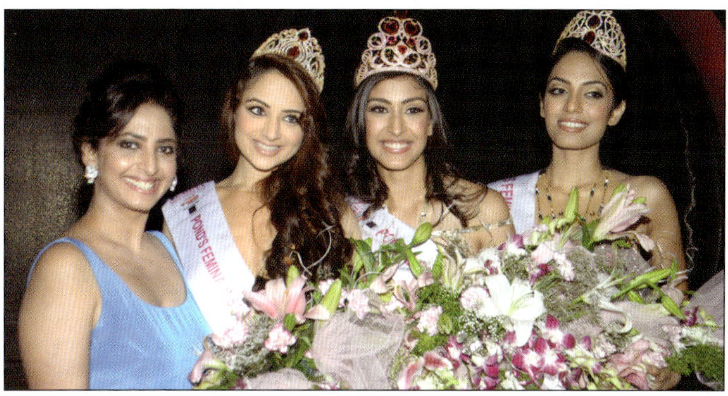

Crowning ceremony with the winners of Femina Miss India 2013, Navneet Kaur Dhillon (M), Shobhita Dhulipala (R), and Zoya Afroz (L)

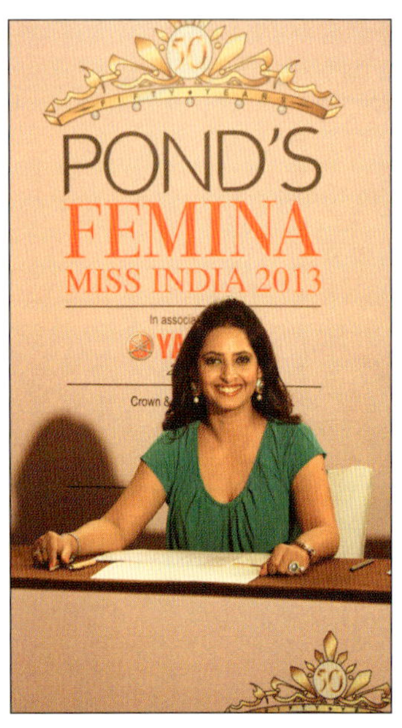

Judging Femina Miss India 2013

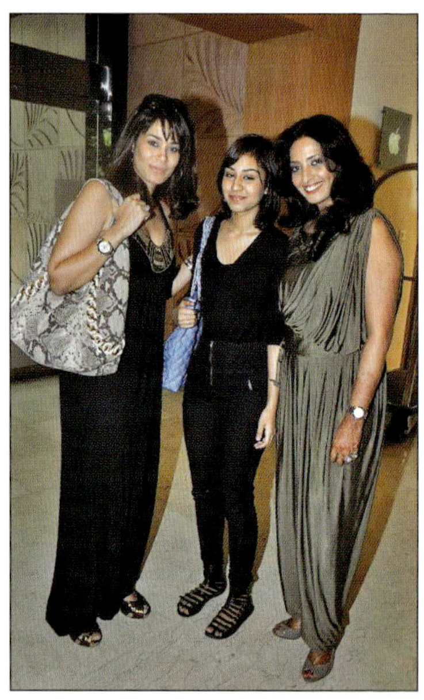

With jewellery designer
Shaheen Abbas (extreme left)

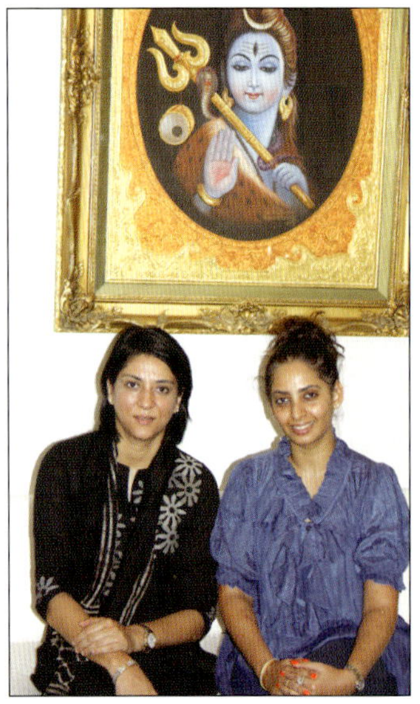

With Priya Dutt

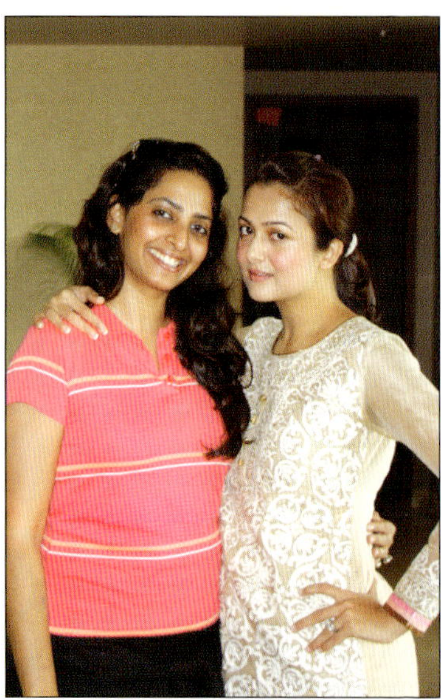

With Amrita Arora Ladak

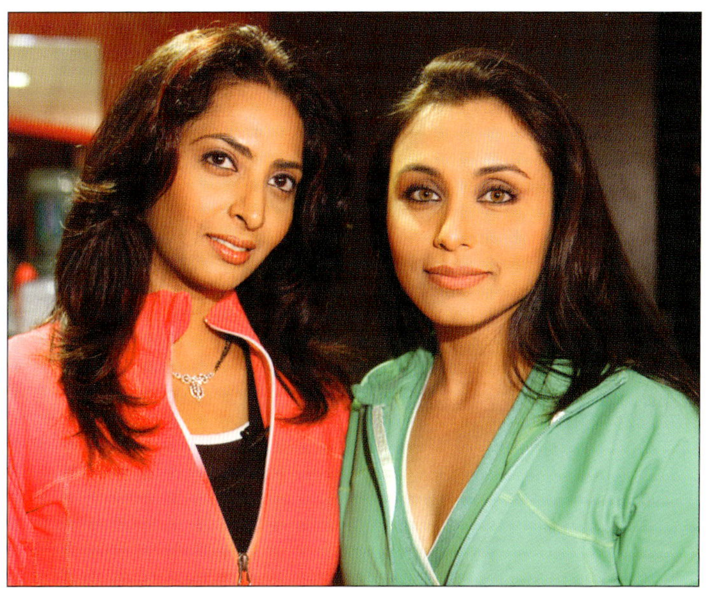

With Rani Mukherji Chopra

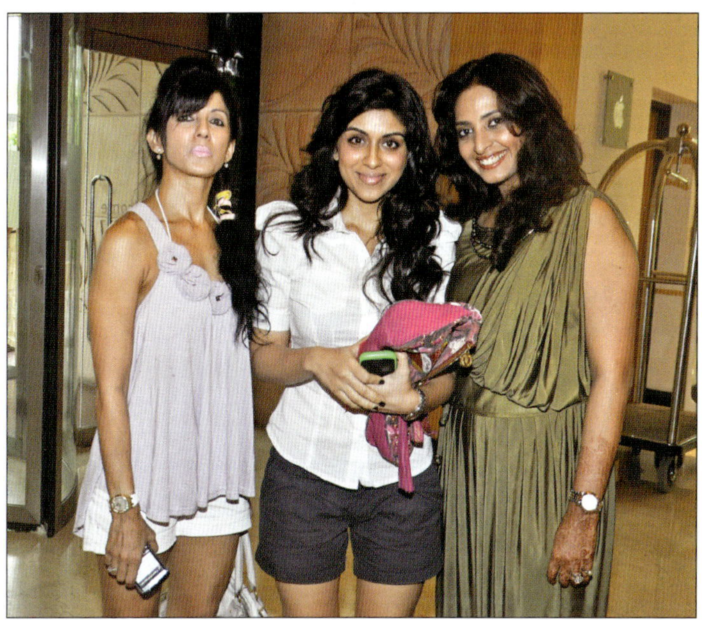

With Actress Zoa Morani (M) and her mother Zara Morani (L)

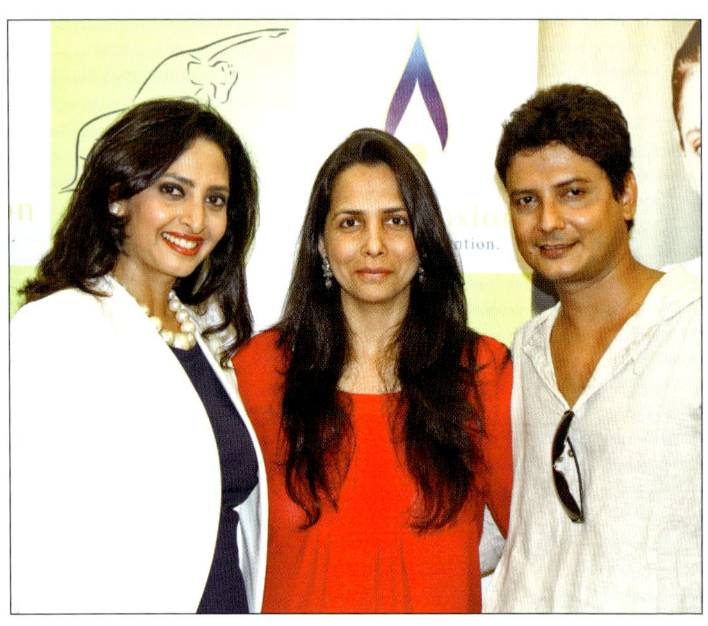

With jewellery designer Roopa Vohra

With theater artists Alyque and Raell Padamsee